A Comprehensive
Model for Children
with Special Needs

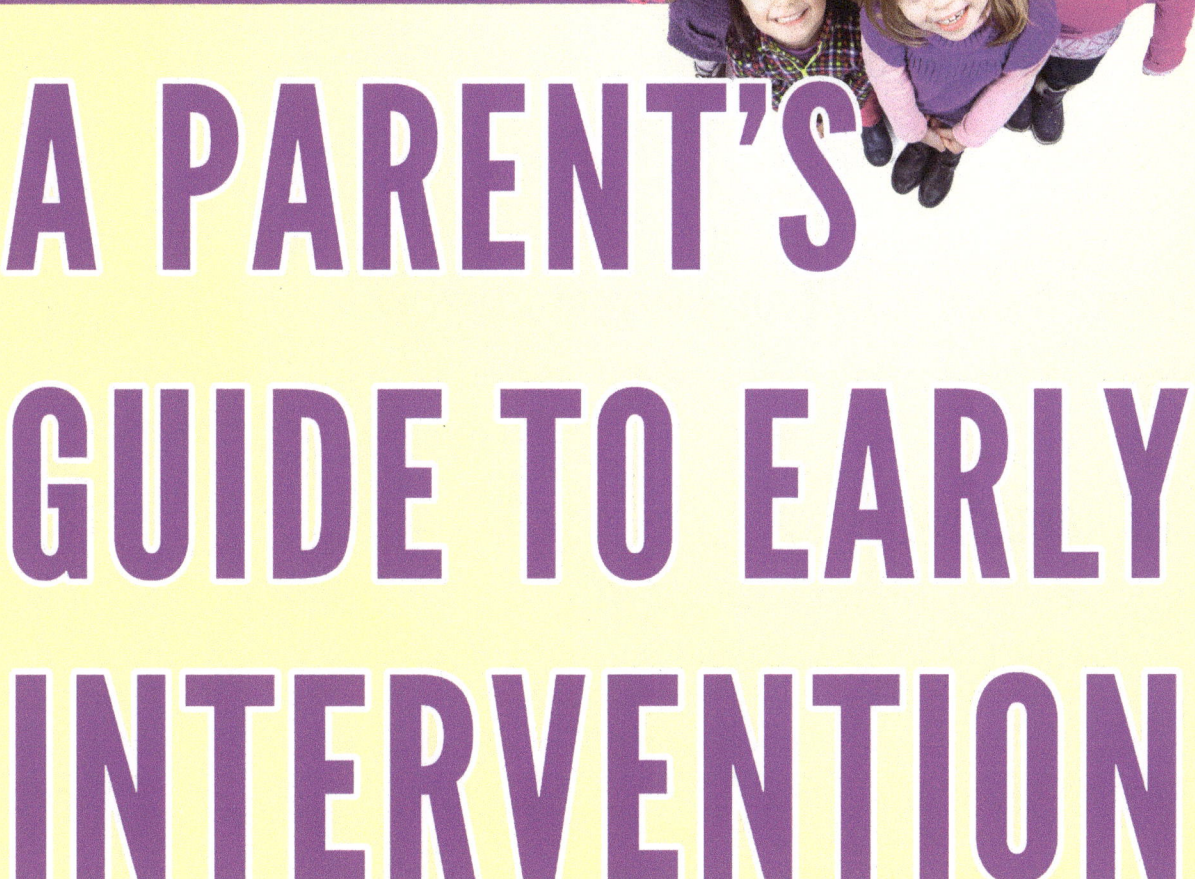

A PARENT'S
GUIDE TO EARLY
INTERVENTION

ALEX LIAU

A PARENT'S GUIDE TO EARLY INTERVENTION

All marketing and publishing rights guaranteed to and reserved by:

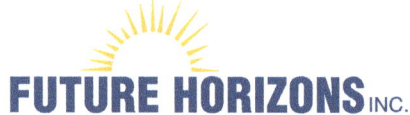

Toll-free: 800·489·0727 | Fax: 817·277·2270

www.FHautism.com | info@FHautism.com

ISBN: 9781949177732

CONTENTS

01   INTRODUCTION 1

02   THE HOME ENVIRONMENT 5

03   EARLY INTENSIVE BEHAVIORAL INTERVENTION. 13

04   FUNCTIONAL SKILLS TRAINING 75

05   SMALL GROUP INTERVENTION 101

06   SCHOOL SHADOW SUPPORT 133

07   SOCIAL SKILLS DEVELOPMENT. 159

08   PARENT SUPPORT. 175

09   CONTINGENCY PLANS 179

10   TRANSITION TO PRIMARY ONE 191

APPENDIX. 201

REFERENCES. 209

Chapter 1

INTRODUCTION

WHAT IS

AUTISM SPECTRUM DISORDER?

Children with Autism Spectrum Disorder (more commonly known as autism) display wide variations in symptoms across the spectrum (National Institute of Mental Health, 2018). Symptoms commonly become apparent to parents before the child turns 2 (NIMH, 2018). While symptoms of autism vary widely across each child, children with autism generally display

1. Social impairments

2. Cognitive impairments

3. Repetitive behaviors (MOH, 2010)

DSM-5

According to DSM-5, the diagnostic criteria of autism are:

1. Persistent deficits in social communication and social interactions across contexts

2. Restricted, repetitive patterns of behavior, interests, or activities

3. Symptoms must be present in early developmental period

4. Symptoms cause significant impairment in social, occupational, or other areas of current functioning

5. These disturbances are not explained by intellectual disability or global developmental delay

INTERVENTION

While there is no cure for autism, several research studies have shown that symptoms of autism can be significantly improved through intervention. For example, research has shown that early intervention for children as young as 18 months have shown to be effective in improving child's cognitive, language and social interaction (Autism Speaks, 2009). Also, an intensive literature review done has also shown that children with autism who went through early intensive behavioral intervention have shown improvements in cognitive improvements, language skills, and adaptive behavior (Warren, Mcpheeters, Sathe, Foss-Feig, 2011).

COMPREHENSIVE MODEL FOR EARLY INTERVENTION

CMEI is a model for autism intervention developed by Alex Liau, Clinical Director of Nurture Pods (Singapore). This model is mainly based on Early Intensive Behavioral Intervention (EIBI), with different strategies based on the stage the child is at. The components of this model have proven effective in past research, targeting all areas of autism from the symptoms of autism to parent and school involvement to provide a more holistic intervention for the child. The different components will be further explained in the later chapters. The different stages are depicted in the figure below. Each component will be further explained in later chapters.

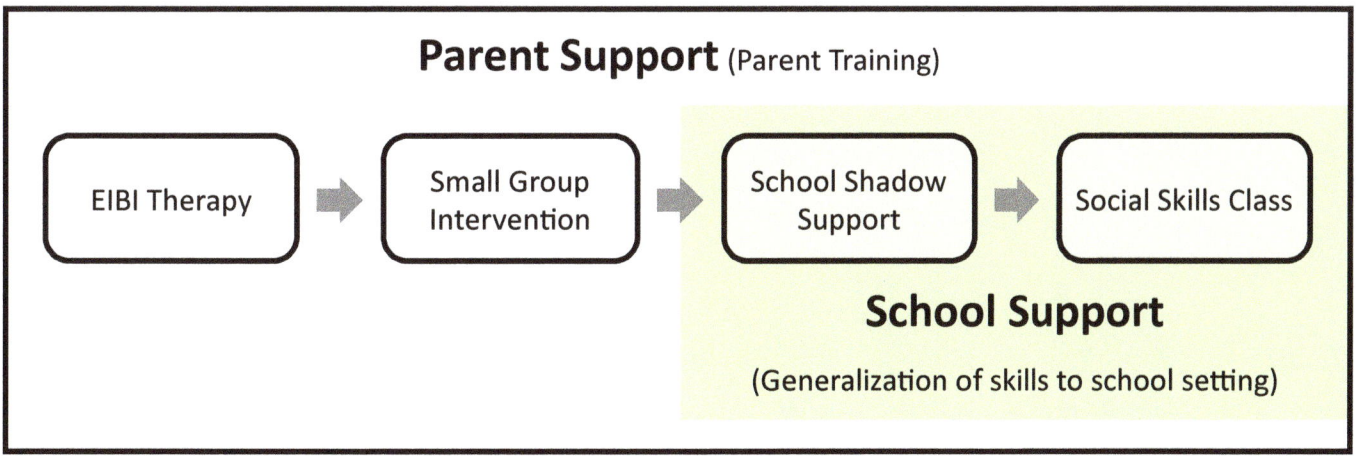

Chapter 2

THE HOME ENVIRONMENT

"CREATING THE BEST ENVIRONMENT FOR YOUR CHILD TO THRIVE IN"

Before looking into intensive intervention for the child, it is important to first look at the home environment and make necessary changes to provide a safe and structured environment for the child. In the environment that best suits the child, the child with autism can thrive.

SENSORY-FRIENDLY ENVIRONMENTS

According to a report by National Autism Network (2016), nearly 90% of children on the autism spectrum face sensory issues such as hypersensitivity in one or more of their senses. Therefore, they may have trouble coping in certain environments, and seemingly small triggers may overwhelm them. So, it is crucial to create a sensory-friendly environment based on your child's needs.

TO CREATE A SENSORY-FRIENDLY ENVIRONMENT

1 **Find out child's sensory needs**

→ What triggers my child's meltdowns?

→ What does my child often reject?

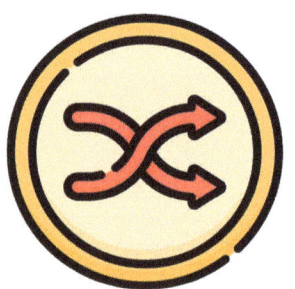

Make changes to house environment **2**

→ Removing/reducing triggering stimulus

3 **Observe outcome**

→ Is my child calmer now?

→ Is my child still displaying signs of meltdown?

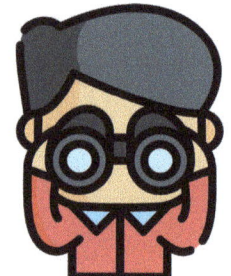

Maintain/Adjust **4**

→ If child is still anxious, try adjusting or making other changes to see it works.

MAKING ADJUSTMENTS TO HOME ENVIRONMENT

	TRIGGER	SUGGESTED ADJUSTMENTS
Sound	**Environmental noises** (e.g., thunder, car sirens)	→ Soundproof windows → Choose room away from roads as child's room
	Household noises (e.g., vacuum cleaner, telephone ringing)	→ Get child to wear headphones → Remove telephone from child's room
Sight	**Bright lights**	→ Light with "dimmer mode" to adjust the brightness of the light according to child's needs (National Autism Network, 2016) → Creative ways of lighting, e.g., fairy lights, night lights (National Autism Network, 2016)
	Colors	→ Low-toned, muted colors for walls with minimal patterns (National Autism Network, 2016)
	Environmental lights (e.g., lightning, street lights)	→ Blackout curtains (National Autism Network, 2016)
Smell	**Strong smells** (e.g., perfumes, air fresheners)	→ Minimize the use of perfumes and air fresheners in the house

USE OF ROUTINES

- To guide a child with ASD in learning appropriate home routines, parents create step-by-step visual routines.

- Routines are especially useful for children with ASD, as it taps on their desires for sameness, which helps them learn routines quickly.

- Routines can be created for tasks that the child must do every day, such as a morning routine, mealtime routine, or bedtime routine.

- As children with ASD are highly visual learners, it is important to have step-by-step pictures for the child to follow.

EXAMPLE OF MORNING ROUTINE

1	Wake up	
2	Use toilet	
3	Brush teeth	
4	Wash face	

USE OF DAILY SCHEDULES

- Daily schedules can help reduce the child's anxiety and increase compliance with tasks.

- Consistent use of the schedule board allows the child to understand

- what is going to happen, giving him a greater sense of predictability.

- This way, the child might be more willing to go through all tasks for the day.

EXAMPLE OF DAILY SCHEDULE

1	**Morning routine**	6	**Read storybooks**
2	**Eat breakfast**	7	**Play time**
3	**Do work**	8	**Eat dinner**
4	**Stretching exercises**	9	**Shower**
5	**Eat lunch**	10	**Sleep**

USE OF VISUAL CALENDARS

- One key importance of having a routine, schedule, and calendar is that it helps the child with autism establish a sense of predictability. Visual calendars help prepare children for activities out of normal routines (e.g., outings, haircut).

- A few days or weeks before the event, parents can write the event down on the calendar and bring it to the child's attention.

- This way, the child knows that something out of routine is going to happen, mitigating their meltdown when presented with the activity.

EXAMPLE OF VISUAL CALENDARS

FEB						
SUN	MON	TUES	WED	THURS	FRI	SAT
1 Church	2 School	3 School	4 School	5 School	6 School	7
8 Church	9 School	10 School	11 School	12 School	13 School	14 Swimming
15 Church	16 School	17 School	18 School	19 School	20 School	21
22 Church	23 HOLIDAY	24 School	25 School	26 School	27 School	28

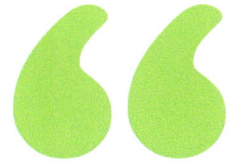

If they can't learn the way we teach, teach the way they learn.

DR. O. IVAR LOVAAS

Chapter 3

EARLY INTENSIVE BEHAVIORAL INTERVENTION

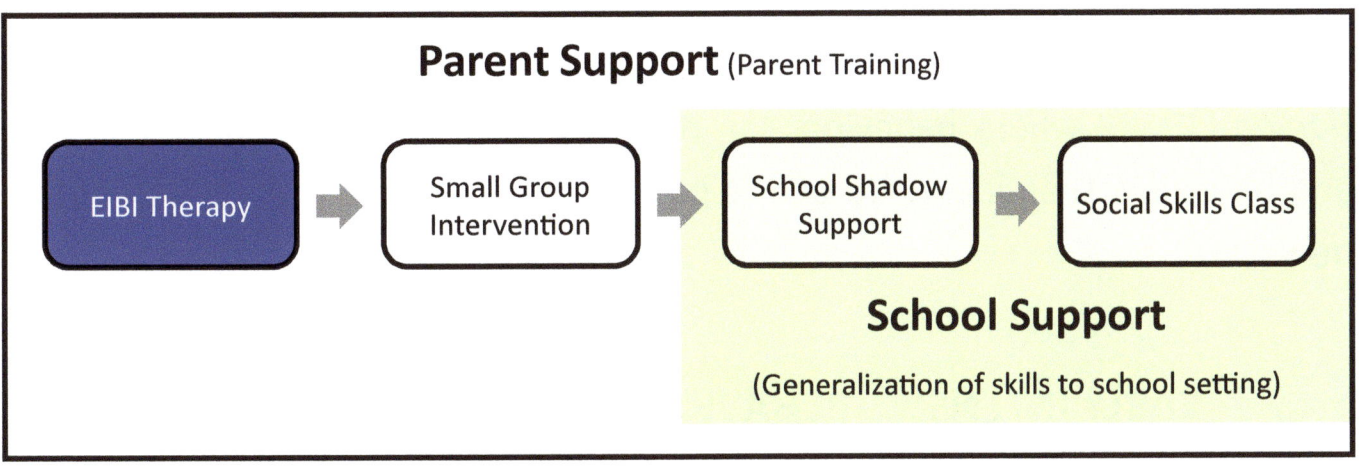

FIRST STAGE OF CMEI MODEL

TARGETING CHILDREN AGES 3-5 YEARS OLD

LARGELY BASED ON APPLIED BEHAVIORAL ANALYSIS (ABA)

HIST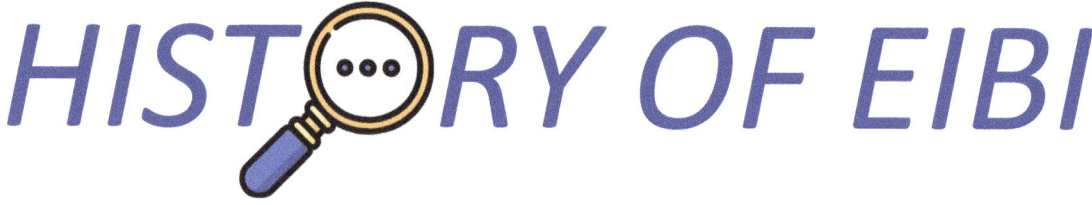RY OF EIBI

APPLIED BEHAVIORAL ANALYSIS (ABA)

ABA is a form of therapy that uses the concepts of learning and motivation to improve good behaviors and skills and decrease inappropriate behaviors (Baer, Wolf & Risley, 1968). It is largely based on B.F. Skinner's *Theory of Operant Conditioning* (1938), where behaviors can be learned based on its consequences, and behaviors that are reinforced (e.g., rewards) are very likely to be continued.

EARLY INTENSIVE BEHAVIORAL INTERVENTION (EIBI)

EIBI encompasses the motivation theory from ABA as well as other important areas that are also important for children's learning, such as behavioral interventions, structured intensive learning in the various domains (e.g., communication, language, numeracy, motor skills, visuospatial skills, and social skills), and support from parents and teachers.

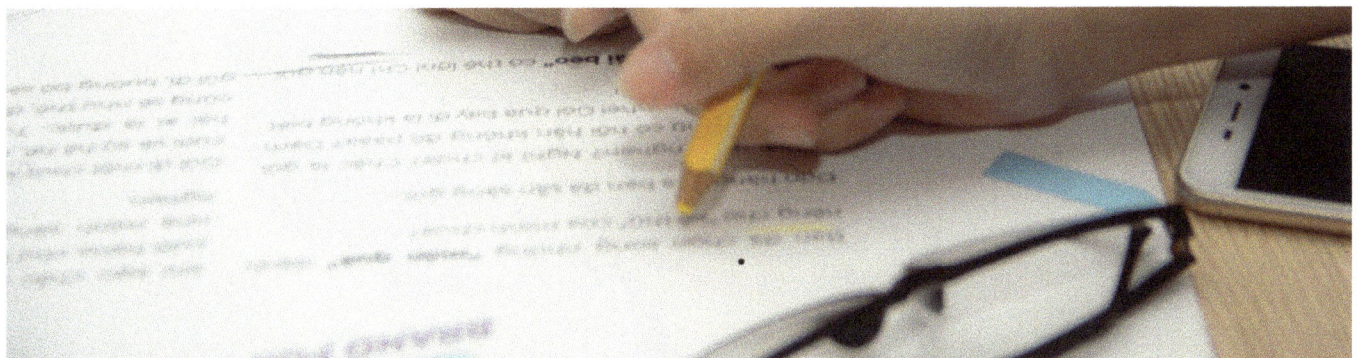

CREATING AN OPTIMAL SPACE FOR THERAPY

→ **Environment free of distractions**

- Find a quiet room in the house
- Find a place with little movement of people
- No distractions—no television, toys, etc.

→ **Appropriate furniture for child**

- Child's table and chair: Child's feet should touch the floor; if not, place a stool under child's feet
- Do **NOT** use adult furniture

→ **Table free of clutter**

- Table should only have:
  1. Token economy
  2. Task Schedule
  3. Task the child is doing

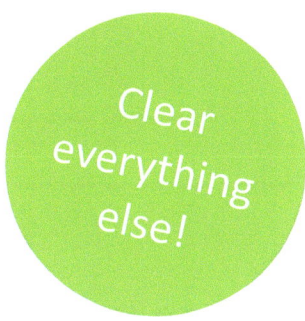

Clear everything else!

TOOLS FOR EIBI

When conducting EIBI, the following tools create structure for the child and act as reinforcements for child's good behaviors. Therefore, it is important for the adult conducting therapy to use all the tools.

1. TOKEN ECONOMY

- The token economy is a reward system that reinforces the child's good behaviors.

- When the child reaches a certain number of tokens (e.g., stars, checkmarks), a reward is given to the child.

- Reward should be kept exclusive to therapy sessions. Child should not receive the reward in any circumstances outside of therapy sessions.

EXAMPLE OF TOKEN ECONOMY

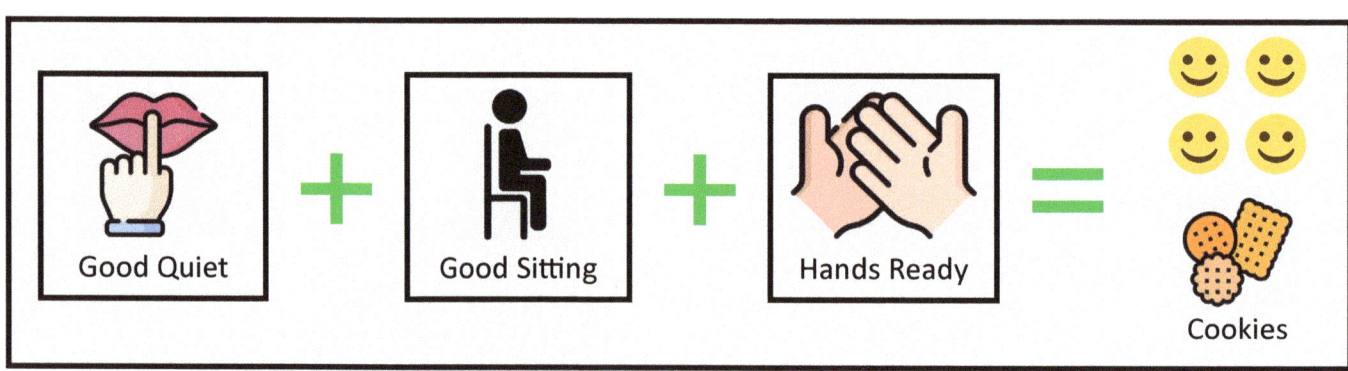

EFFECTIVENESS OF TOKEN ECONOMY

Research has found evidence for the effectiveness of token economy on children with special needs. Two examples of the findings are as follows:

- With the use of token economy, children with special needs successfully learned various good behaviors such as remaining in their seat for therapy. Token economy also boosts children's attention to tasks (Matson & Boisjoli, 2009)

- Token economy is effective in correcting challenging behaviors in a child with autism, especially when rewards are in-line with the child's interests (Carneet et al., 2014)

COMPONENTS OF TOKEN ECONOMY

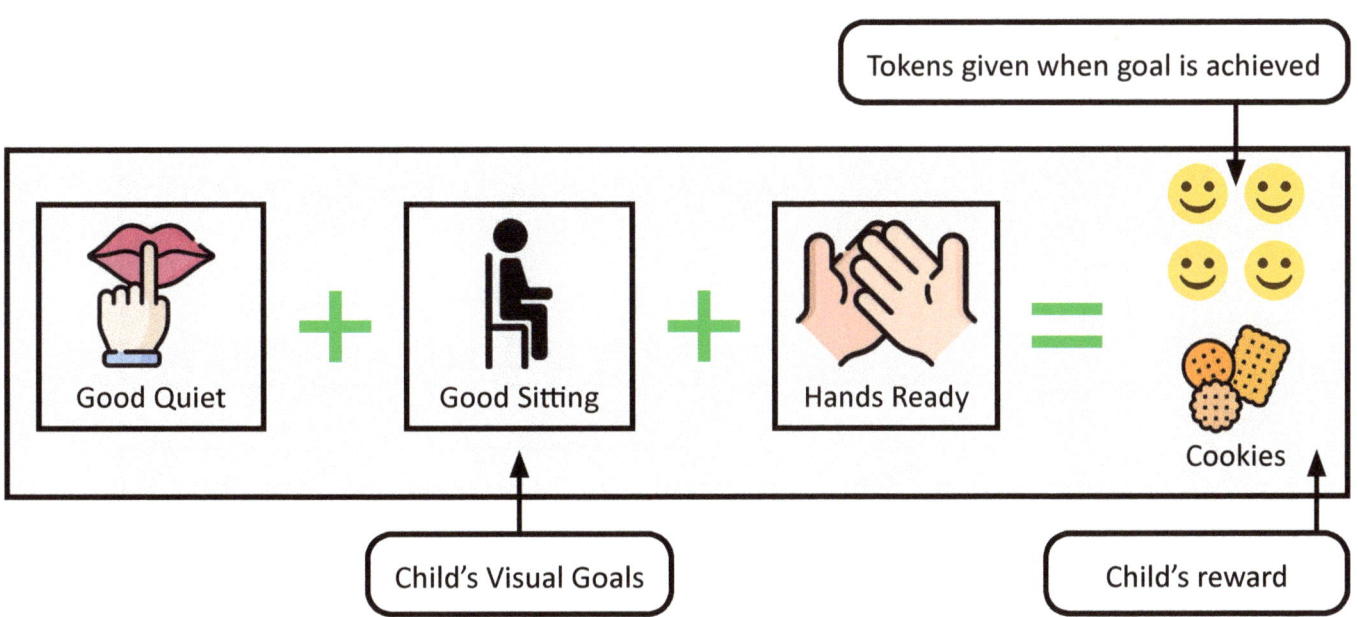

HOW TO USE TOKEN ECONOMY*

1 **Decide on goals and reward.**

List of possible goals in Appendix
Guidelines for choosing rewards on Page 20

2 **Explain to child the goals and rewards, pointing to each component when explaining**

E.g., " If you show good sitting, good quiet and good hands ready, you get a smiley! With four smileys, you earn a cookie!"

3 **Whenever child reaches a goal, give child a token. Be sure to let child know why he is earning the token!**

E.g., "Very good sitting! You get one smiley!"

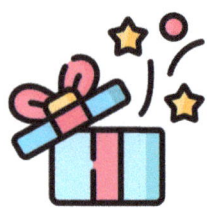 

4 **When child earns a token, he gets the reward. Be sure to let child know why he is getting the reward!**

E.g., "Look, you earned 4 smileys (Count the smileys with the child). Here is your cookie!)

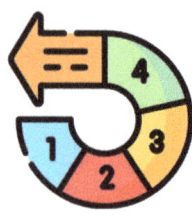 

5 **Restart the token economy by removing all smileys. Repeat steps 3-5 until the end of the session.**

* For token economy to be effective, it must be used consistently!

TOKEN ECONOMY TIPS

1. **Do NOT bribe or threaten the child, as it makes them reliant on rewards**

   ➜ Examples:

   ✖ "If you sit, then I will give you a token"

   ✖ "If you make noise, then I will take away the token"

2. **Do NOT reinforce with tokens immediately after prompting child for good behaviors**

   ➜ Examples:

   ✔ If child keeps quiet after you tell them to keep quiet, do not give a token immediately for "good quiet" as the behavior was prompted. Instead, you can praise them for listening well to your instructions.

   ✔ Tokens should only be given when child displays good behaviors **without prompts.**

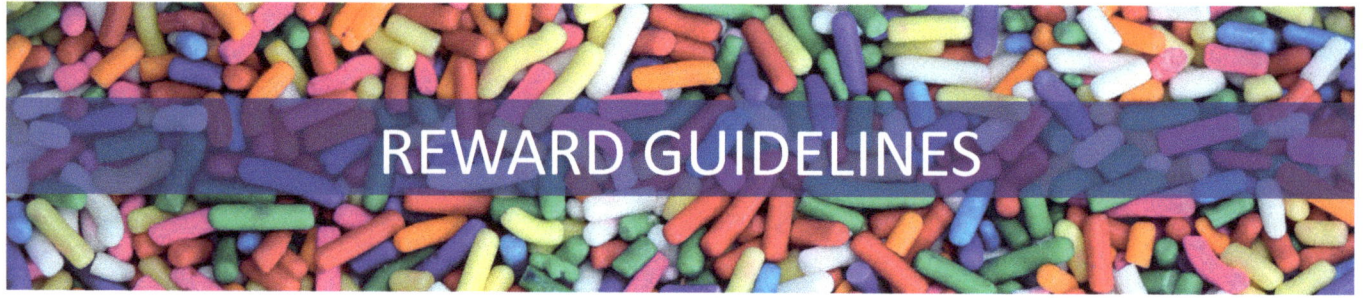

REWARD GUIDELINES

CHOOSING A REWARD

Reward should be small and easily given yet rewarding for the child.

- Better if administering of the reward does not take too much time, such that when the child gets the reward in the middle of the session, he is able to go back to the tasks quickly

- E.g., M&Ms, jellybeans

Reward should be kept **exclusive**

- Choose rewards that the child does not need to have on a regular basis, such that the reward can only be given in therapy sessions.

REWARD HIERARCHY

- Initially, tokens should be given every 5-10 seconds to allow the child to understand the reward system.

- Slowly wean off to every 4-5 minutes per token

- After child can display good behaviors with that frequency, start giving tokens inconsistently (e.g., sometimes every 10 seconds, sometimes after 10 minutes)

- Reward should start from **food** (e.g., cookie), followed by **toys** (e.g., bubbles) and then weaned off to **praises** (e.g., high-5s, "good job!")

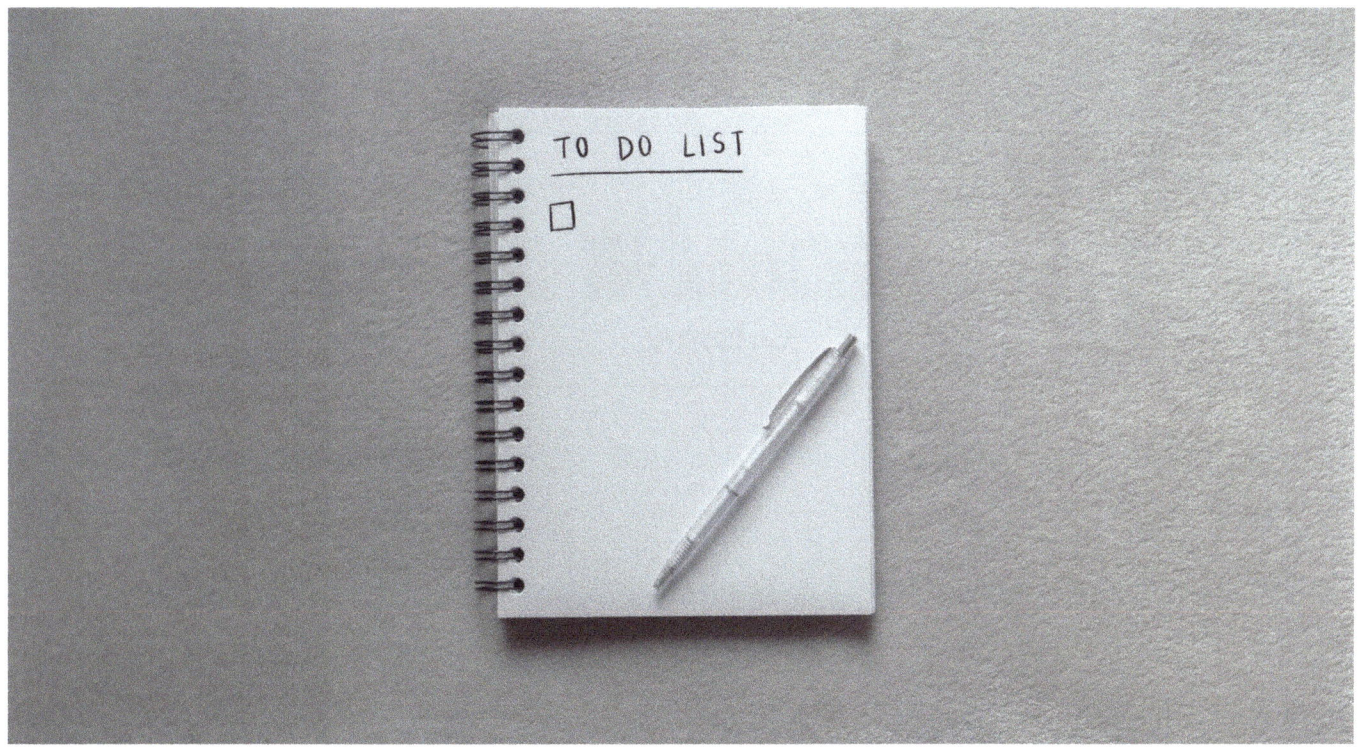

2. Task Schedules

For children with autism, schedules are very important as they help them be aware of what is going to happen, reducing their anxiety. Having a schedule also creates structure in the intervention sessions, and as children with ASD thrive better in a structured environment, schedules help the child focus and calm down. Parents of children with ASD also often report that their child tends to be more compliant with doing the tasks with the use of a schedule.

EXAMPLE OF TASK SCHEDULE

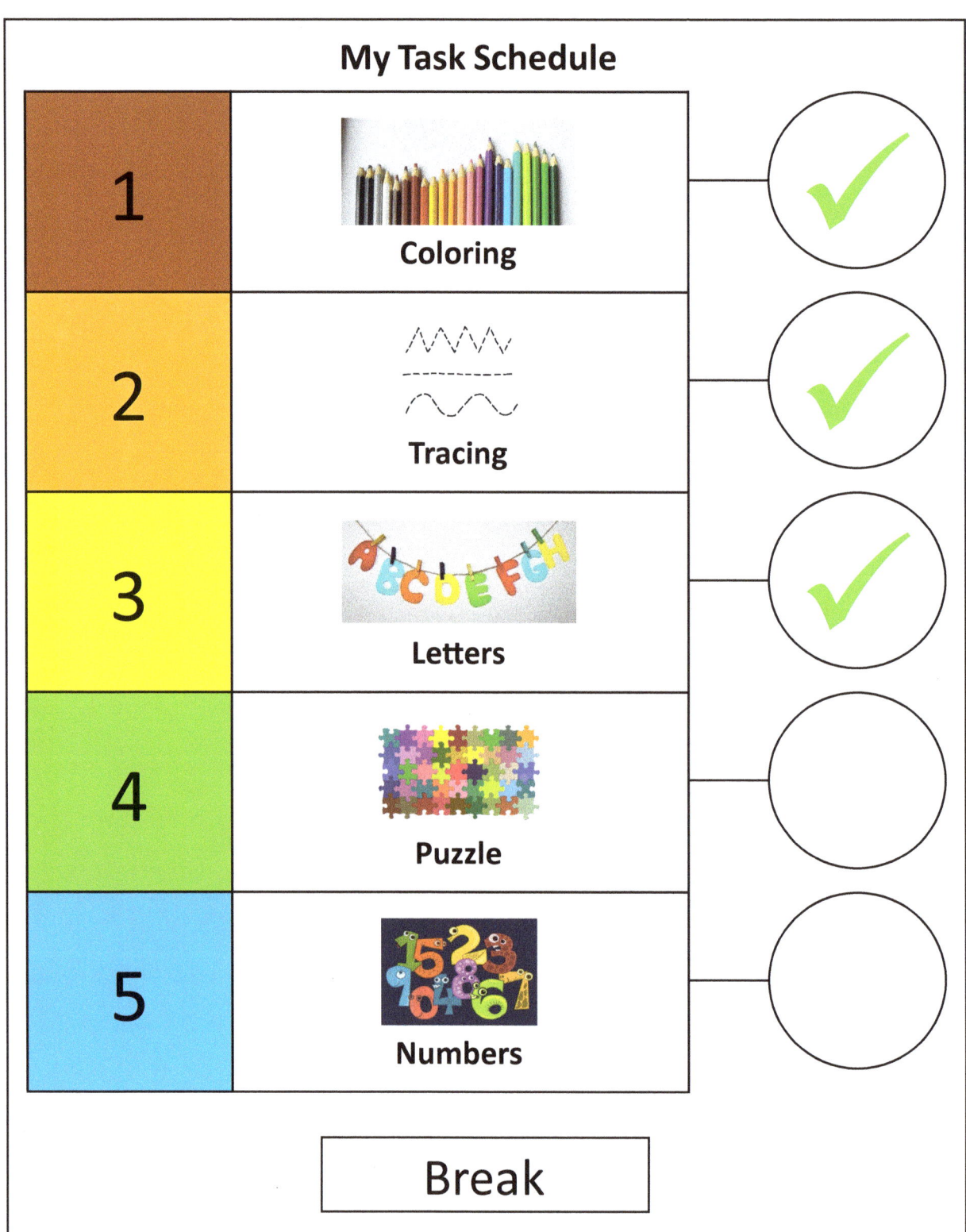

HOW TO USE A TASK SCHEDULE

Decide on tasks and paste tasks on schedule.

Refer to page 24 for tips on task selection and order.

Explain to child what task he needs to complete before he gets a break (while pointing to task)

E.g.," Number 1, we do coloring. Number 2, Tracing. Number 3, Letters. Number 4, puzzle. Number 5, numbers. Then we go for a break!"

When the child completes the task, get the child to paste a checkmark beside the task

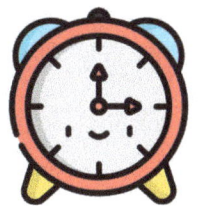 

After child finishes all 5 tasks, he is allowed to go for a break.

E.g., "Numbers 1, 2, 3, 4, 5, all finished! Now you can go for a 5-minute break!"

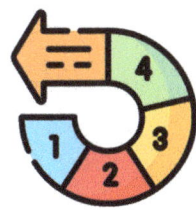 

Set a timer and create a new task schedule. Once timer is up, start a new cycle. Repeat steps 1-5 until the session ends.

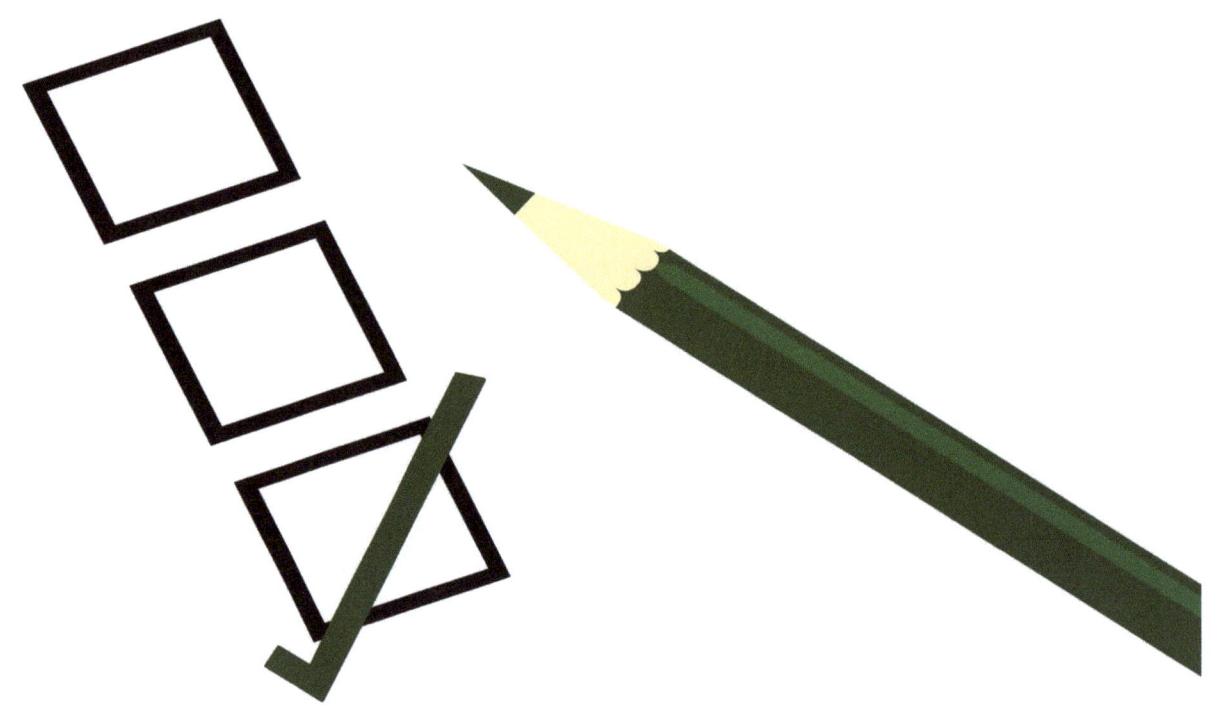

TASK SCHEDULE TIPS

- Number of tasks can differ for each cycle ➜ Do not adhere to a certain number of tasks every cycle as it may create rigidity in the child.

- Choose a number of tasks based on child's abilities and focus, and

- the intensity of the tasks.

- Task schedule must be used **consistently** and placed in a spot where the child can refer to it **all the time.**

- The order of tasks is important. Therapist can create task schedules such that easy and hard tasks are alternated with each other (e.g., 1. Easy task, 2. Hard task, 3. Easy task).

EIBI TASKS

EIBI tasks can generally be targeted in four main areas:

1. Language (literacy) development

2. Cognitive development

3. Motor skills development

4. Visuospatial skills development

Hierarchy of reinforcement for tasks

While good behaviors are reinforced by the token economy, when the child does well in tasks, that should also be reinforced. Below is a guideline to help motivate the child to get the correct answer on the first try.

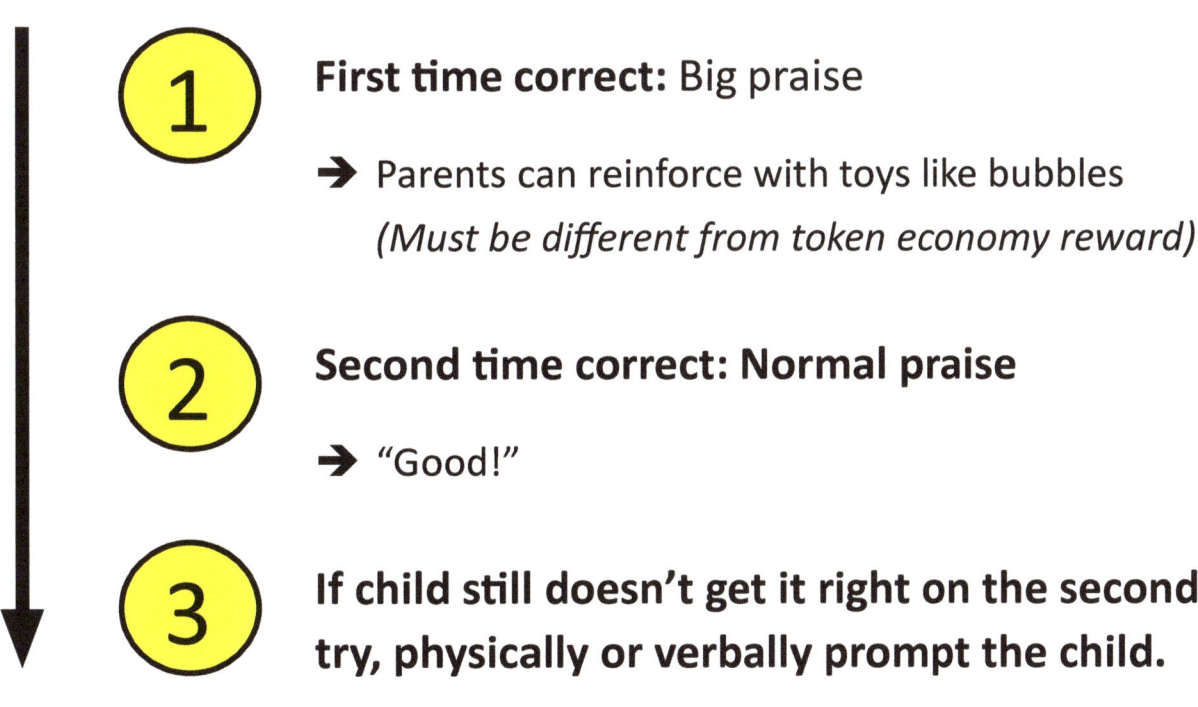

1 **First time correct:** Big praise

➔ Parents can reinforce with toys like bubbles
(Must be different from token economy reward)

2 **Second time correct: Normal praise**

➔ "Good!"

3 **If child still doesn't get it right on the second try, physically or verbally prompt the child.**

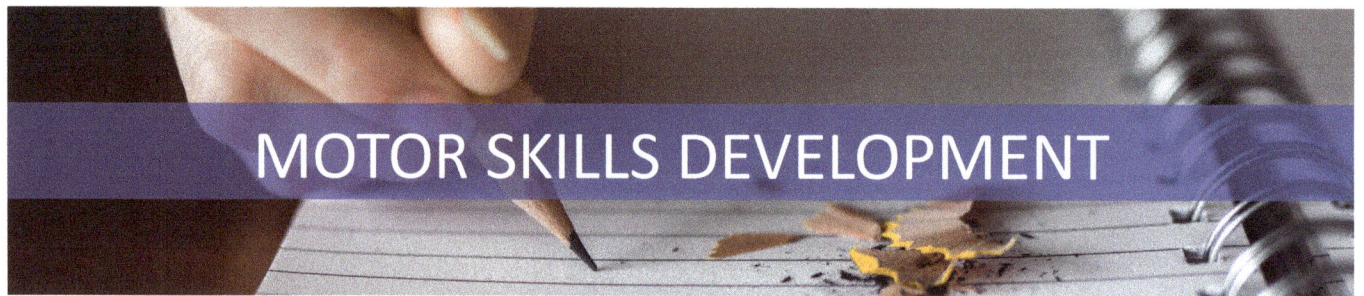

MOTOR SKILLS DEVELOPMENT

Motor skill is a function which involves the precise movement of muscles with the intent to perform a specific act. Most purposeful movements require the ability to "feel" or sense what one's muscles are doing as they perform the act. Motor skills include toileting, dressing, eating, personal self-care, domestic skills, and work skills.

EIBI targets language development based on two main components:

1. Gross motor skills: using legs, arms, etc.

2. Fine motor skills: using hands, fingers, etc.

MOTOR SKILLS DEVELOPMENT

⋯→ *Number concept*

- Goal: Gain an understanding of basic **mathematical concept**

 **Sit on floor/table with the child.**

 **Engage the child by saying their name or touching the child's arm.**

 **After you have the child's attention, say "[child's name], do this." At the same time, perform the action that you are trying to teach.**

 **If child repeats your actions, give reinforcers. If not, repeat step 2 and 3, or hand-over-hand to do the action with the child.**

MOTOR SKILLS DEVELOPMENT

2. *Fine motor skills*

Fine motor skills development focuses on developing finger strength and coordination, which eventually helps the child write, cut, and use various other tools with their hands.

STAGES FOR FINE MOTOR SKILLS DEVELOPMENT

Fine motor skills toys

→ Hiding marbles in theraputty and getting the child to dig it out

→ Threading items through a string

→ Using small tools (e.g., tweezers) to pick up items (e.g., marshmallows)

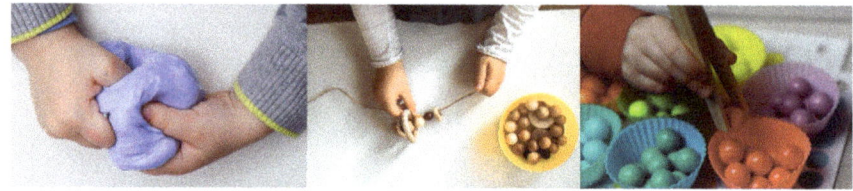

Drawing vertical and horizonal lines on whiteboard.

MOTOR SKILLS DEVELOPMENT

2. *Fine motor skills (continued)*

③

Tracing on paper using marker

→ Stage 1: Horizonal lines

→ Stage 2: Vertical lines

→ Stage 3: Up-down lines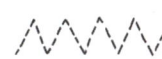

→ Stage 4: Curves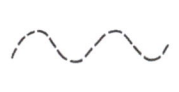

→ Stage 5: Shapes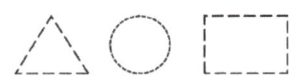

④

Tracing letters and words with pencil and paper
(Hand over hand if necessary)

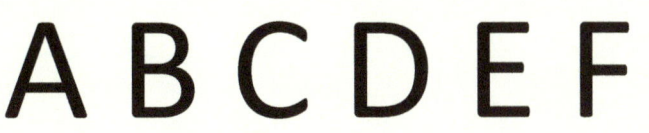

⑤

Copying letters and words
(Hand over hand if necessary)

Child copies
word here!

Hello	

⑥

Cutting paper with scissors

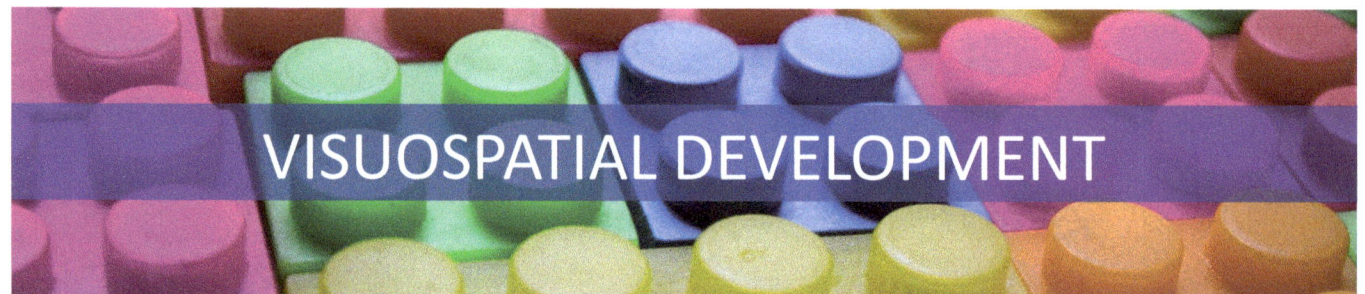

VISUOSPATIAL DEVELOPMENT

- Visuospatial ability refers to a person's capacity to identify visual and special relationships among objects.

- It is measured in terms of the ability to imagine objects, to make global shapes by locating small components, or to understand the differences and similarities between objects.

EIBI encompasses several tasks that help the child's visuospatial development.

Three common tasks are:

1. Number concept

2. Gradation

3. Patterning

VISUOSPATIAL DEVELOPMENT

- Taught with the following stages:

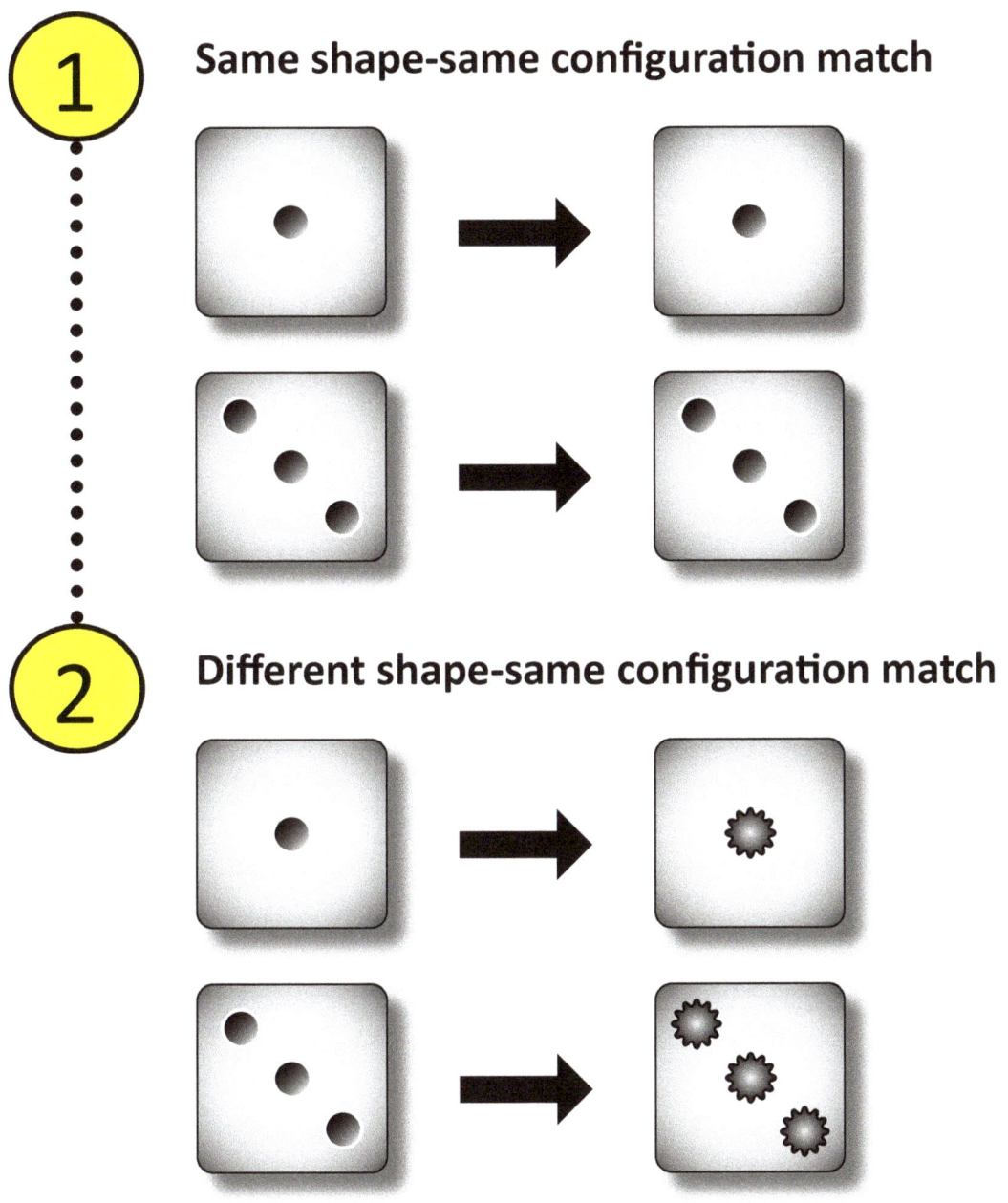

1 Same shape-same configuration match

2 Different shape-same configuration match

VISUOSPATIAL DEVELOPMENT

···→ *Number concept (continued)*

3 **Different shape-different configuration match**

4 **Number (with quantity) and quantity match**

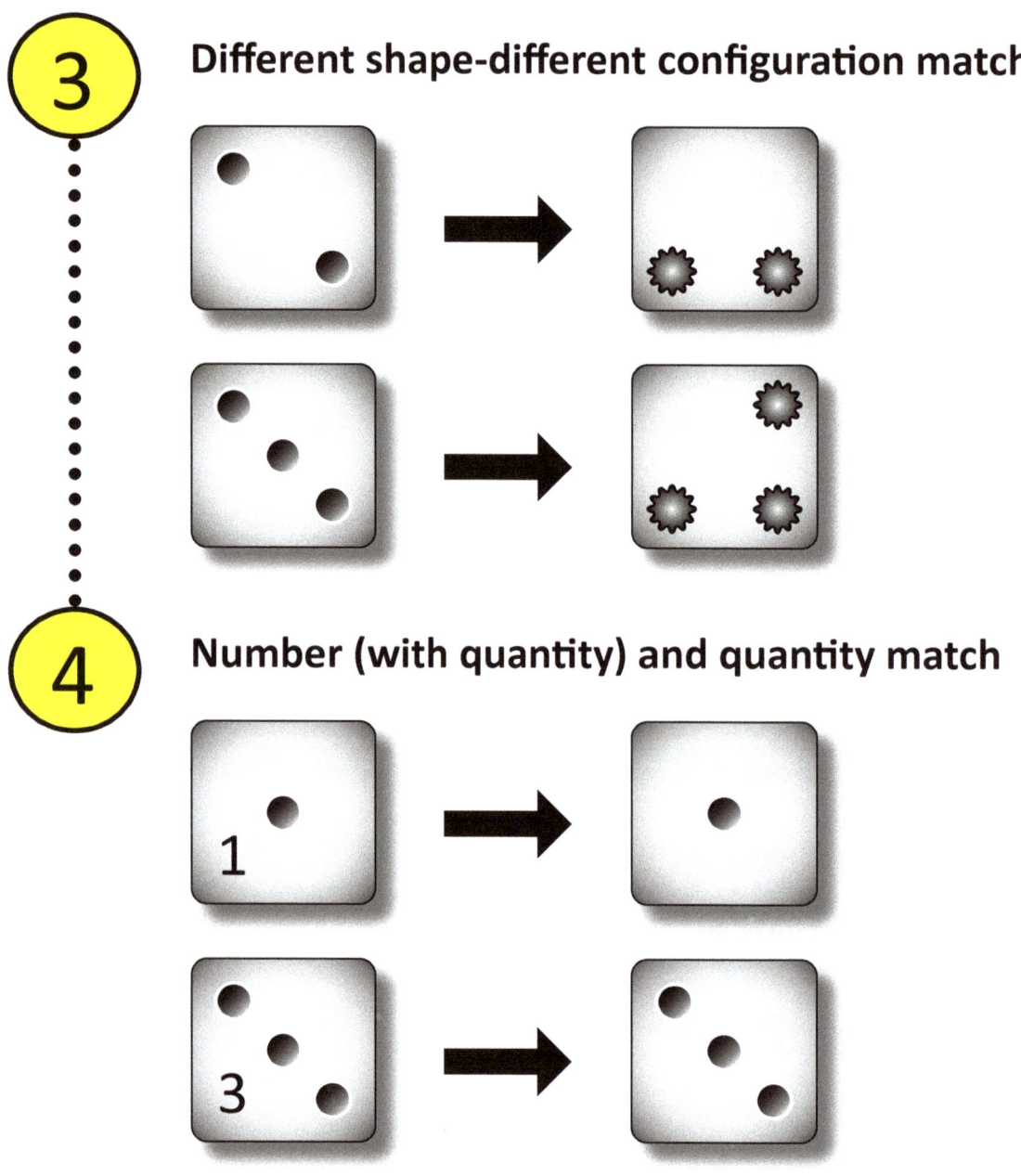

VISUOSPATIAL DEVELOPMENT

⋯→ *Number concept (continued)*

5 **Number and quantity match**

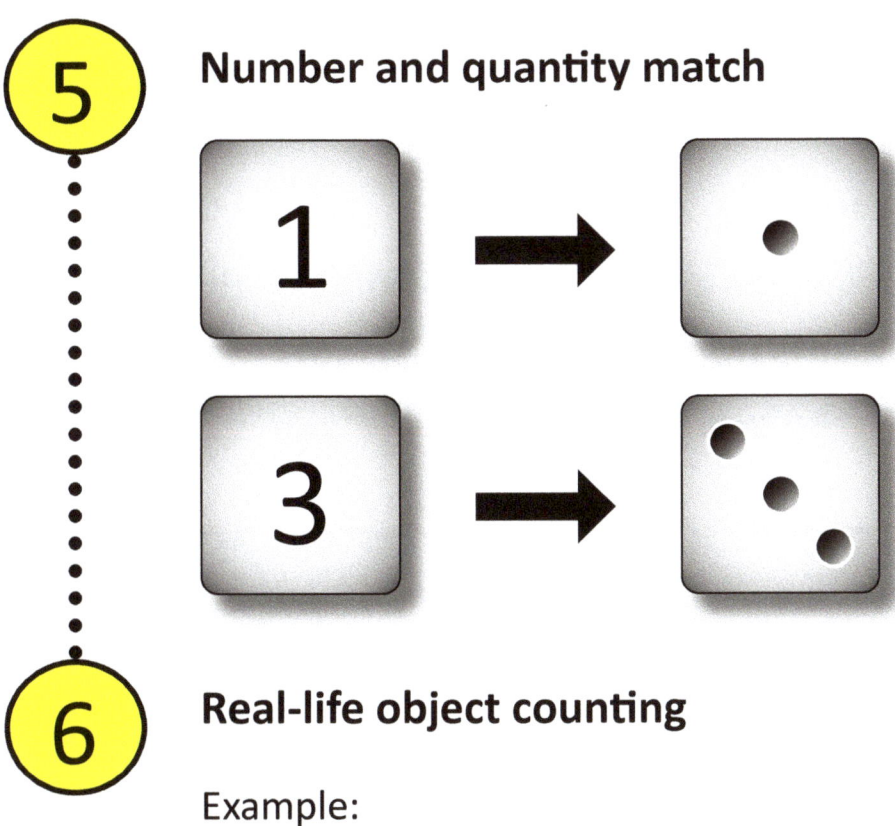

6 **Real-life object counting**

Example:

"Give me 5 pencils"

"Give me 6 sweets"

VISUOSPATIAL DEVELOPMENT

⋯→ *Gradation*

- Goal: Increase the child's understanding and awareness of quantity

Teaching Phase

- Start with 3 cards

- Provide the minimum and maximum quantity on the chart

- Allow child to fill in the intermediate quantity

    Example: "Arrange from small to large"

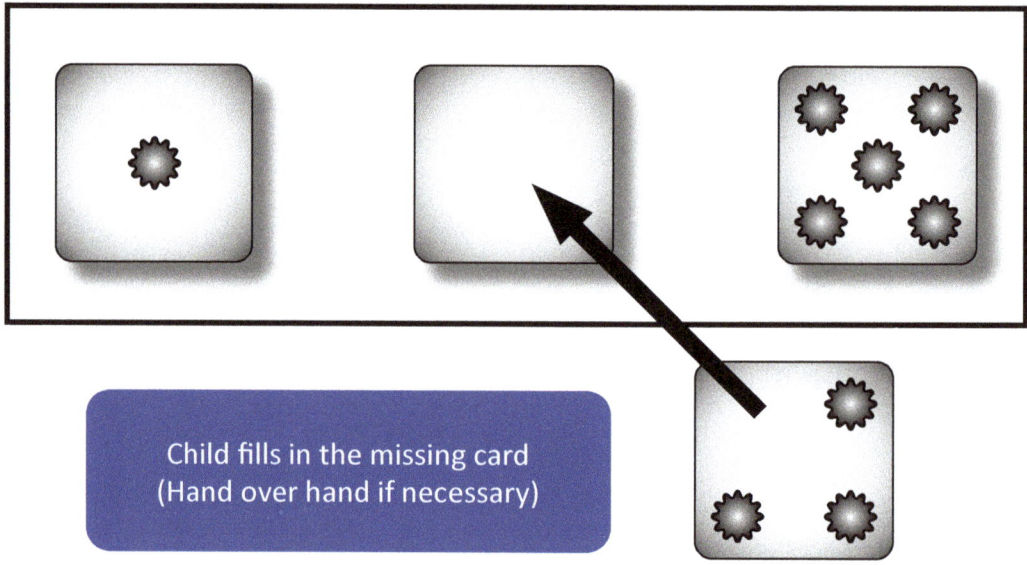

Child fills in the missing card
(Hand over hand if necessary)

VISUOSPATIAL DEVELOPMENT

⋯→ *Gradation (continued)*

- Goal: Increase the child's understanding and awareness of quantity

Practice Phase

- Start with 3 cards, increase to 4-5 cards once child understands concept.

- Increase variations:
    Size – arranging from small to big

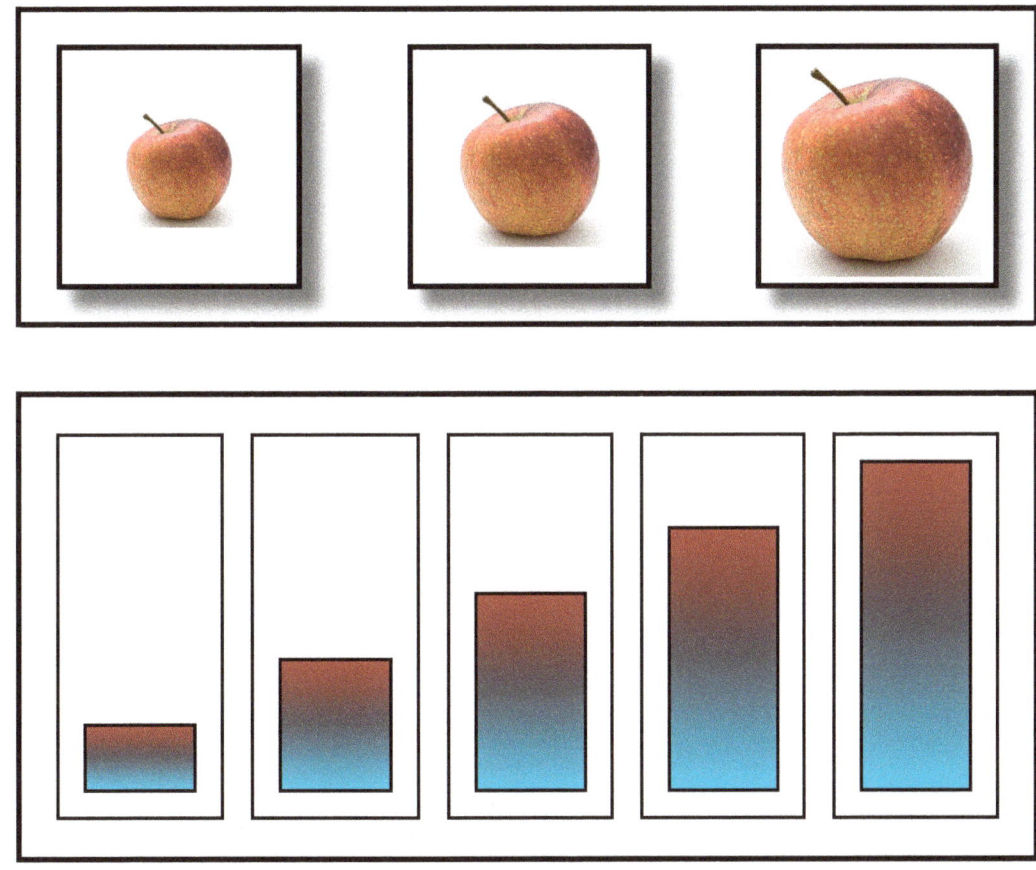

VISUOSPATIAL DEVELOPMENT

⋯→ *Block design*

- Goal: Train child's understanding and awareness in 3D space

1 **Parent builds a block design**

Example:

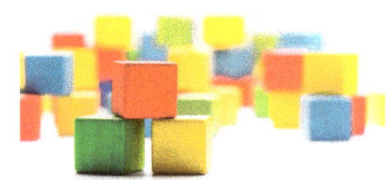

2 **Child receives the exact same blocks and copies the design**

3 **Progress according to the following stages:**

- Stacking
- Side by side
- Hidden blocks
- Extra "unused" blocks for child as distraction

VISUOSPATIAL DEVELOPMENT

⋯→ *Patterning*

- Goal: Train pattern recognition.

Teaching Phase

- Parent completes the first row of the patterning board in front of child, naming the color along the way.

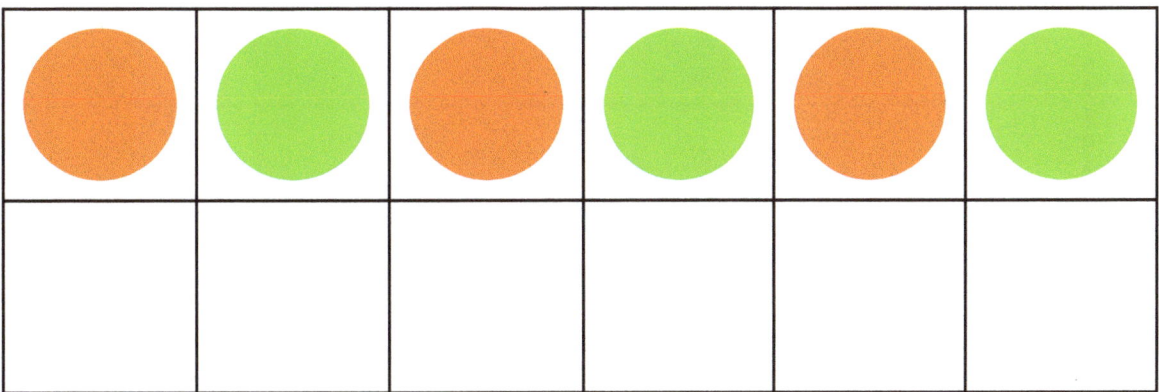

- Parent guides child to do the second row together in the exact ABAB pattern (hand-over-hand if necessary).

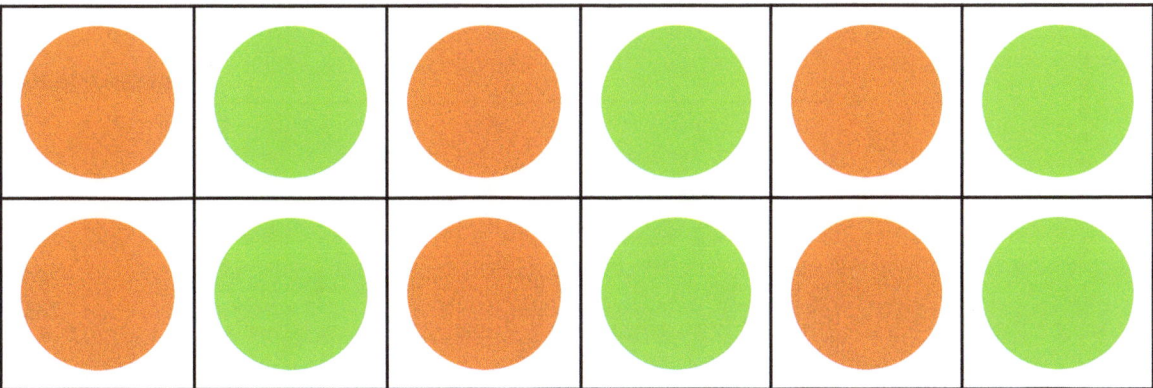

VISUOSPATIAL DEVELOPMENT

⋯→ *Patterning (continued)*

Testing phase 1

- Parent places the first row again; however, this time, remove the last two.

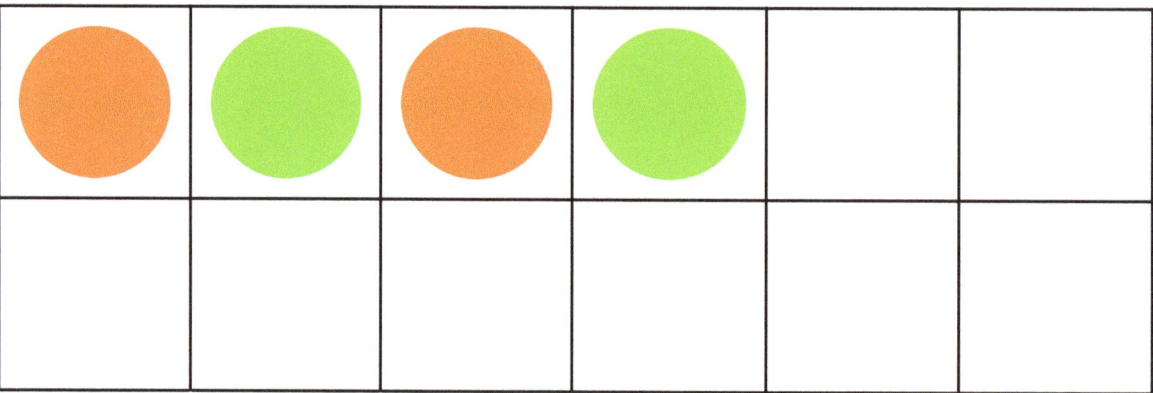

- Child now places the tiles onto the second row from the beginning to the last box.

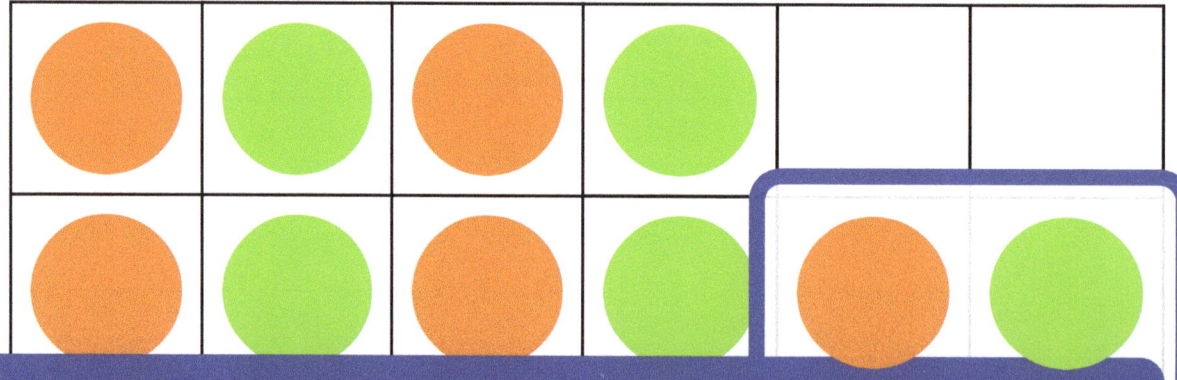

For these two, the child should not have prompts to refer to. Therefore, if the child gets it right, he is starting to understand patterns.

VISUOSPATIAL DEVELOPMENT

···→ *Patterning (continued)*

Testing phase 2

- Now, parents only place the first 2 tiles on the board.

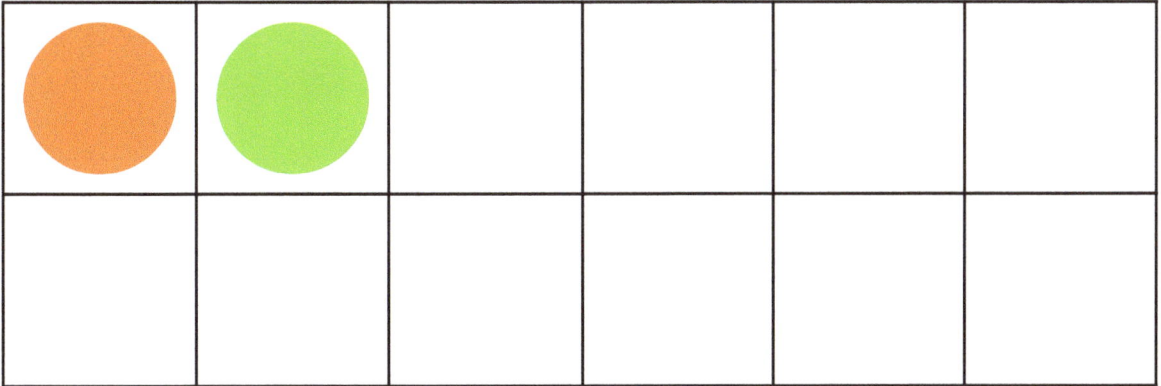

- Child now places the tiles on the second row from the first to the last box.

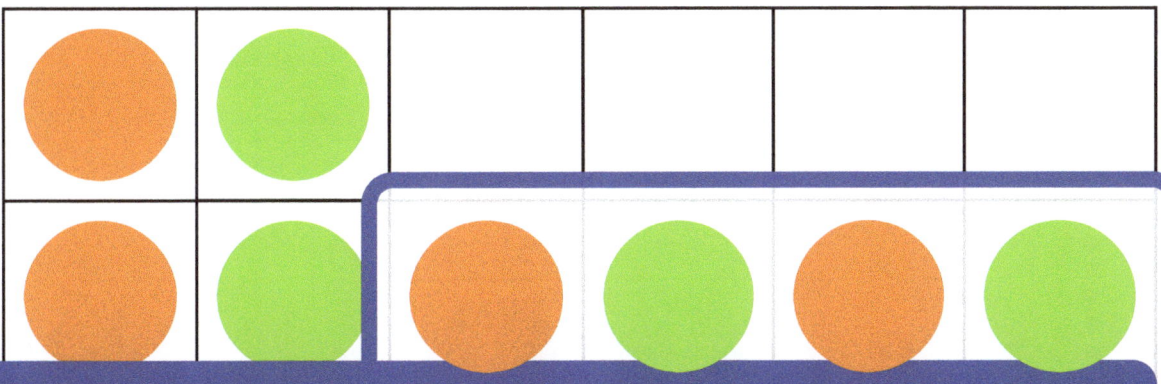

These 4 are now without prompt. If the child gets it, he has a good understanding of patterns. If he doesn't get it, do hand-over-hand with him or go back to previous stages.

VISUOSPATIAL DEVELOPMENT

⋯→ *Patterning (continued)*

Other variations

- Once the child masters the basic ABAB patterning, parents can move on to other variations, using the exact same steps:

ABBABB patterns

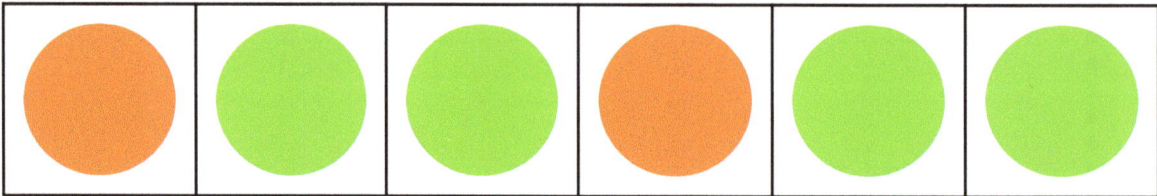

AABAAB patterns

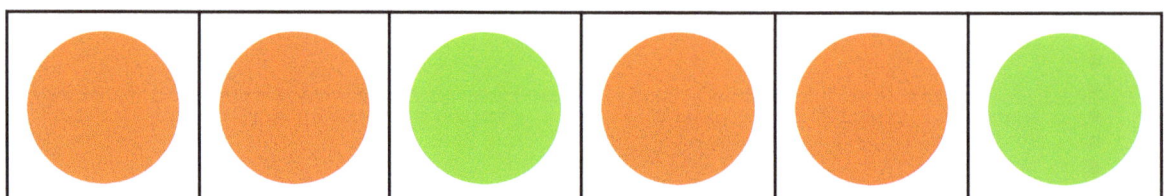

ABCABC patterns

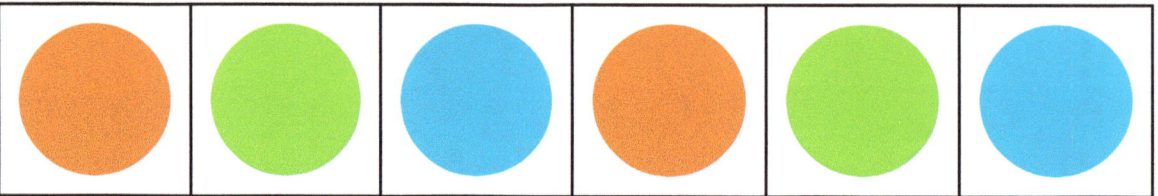

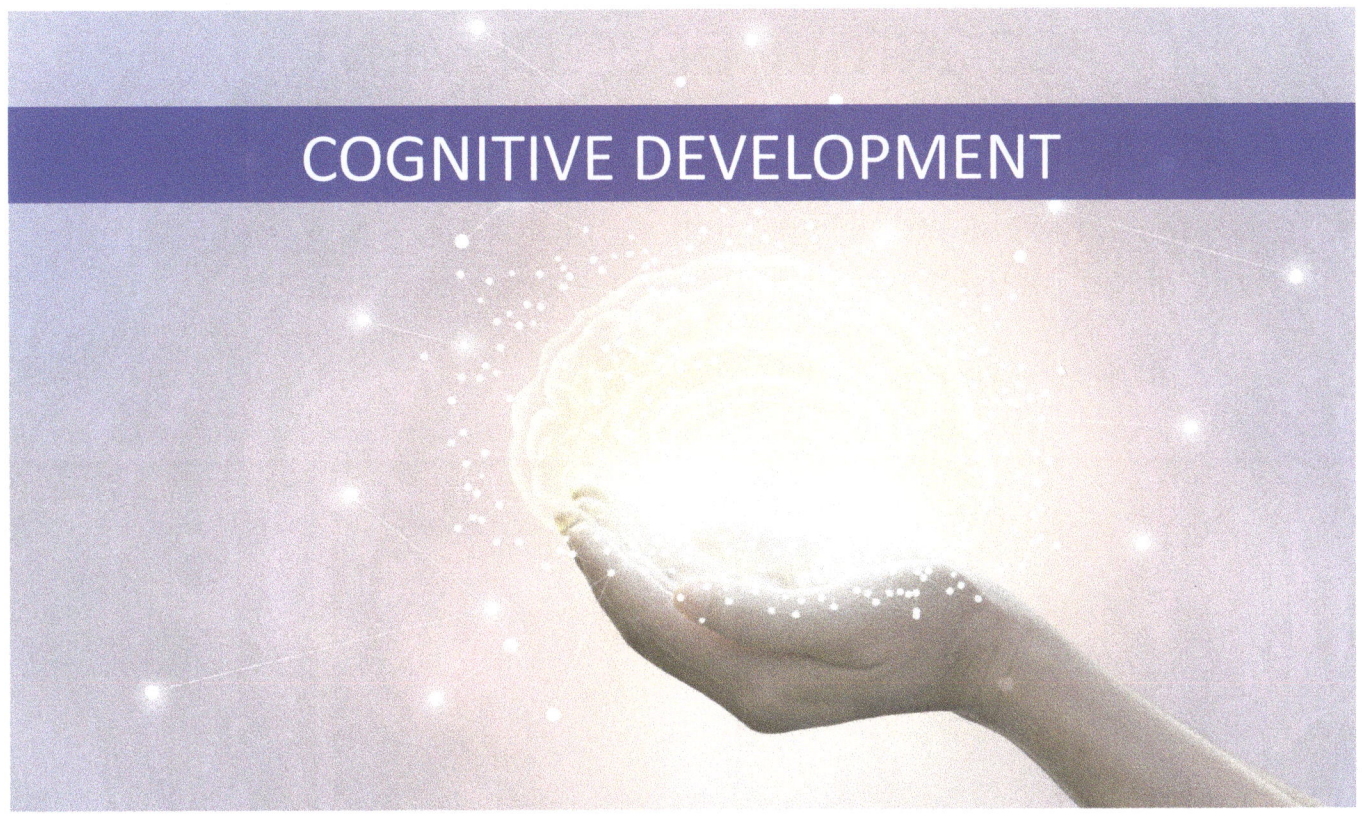

Cognitive skills are crucial to develop a child's reasoning and conceptual ability in the child's later years. EIBI targets cognitive skills development with the following tasks:

1. Part-whole puzzle

2. Follow the rule

COGNITIVE DEVELOPMENT

⸱⸱⸱➔ *Part-Whole Puzzle*

- Goal: Teach the child to recognize that a puzzle piece represents part of a whole object, developing the child's representational skills.

What is needed?

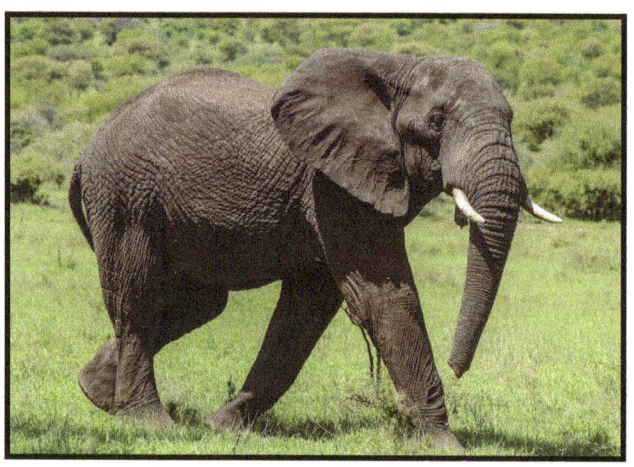

Full picture card

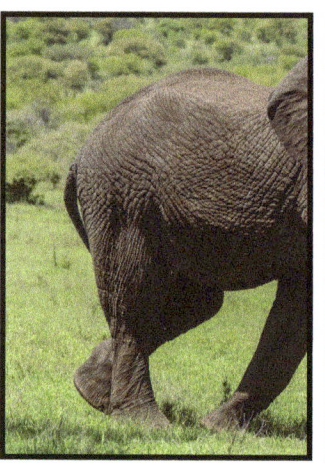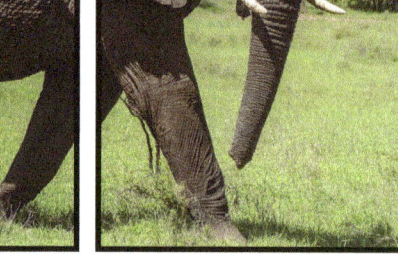

Picture card divided to two parts

Variations for cutting the picture

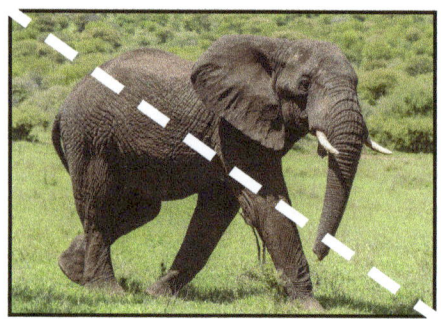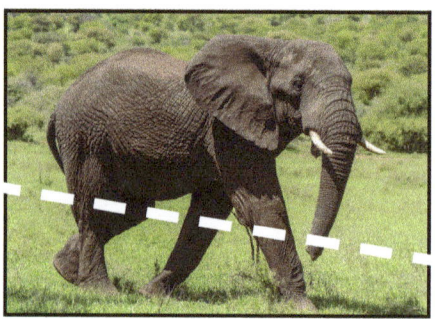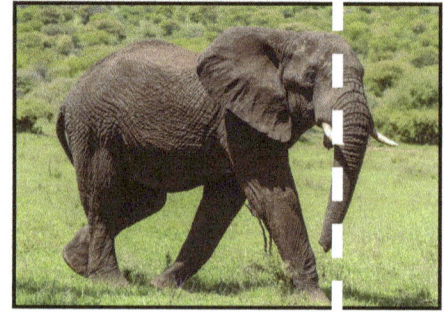

COGNITIVE DEVELOPMENT

···→ *Part-Whole Puzzle (continued)*

How can I do part-whole?

Display the full picture on the table

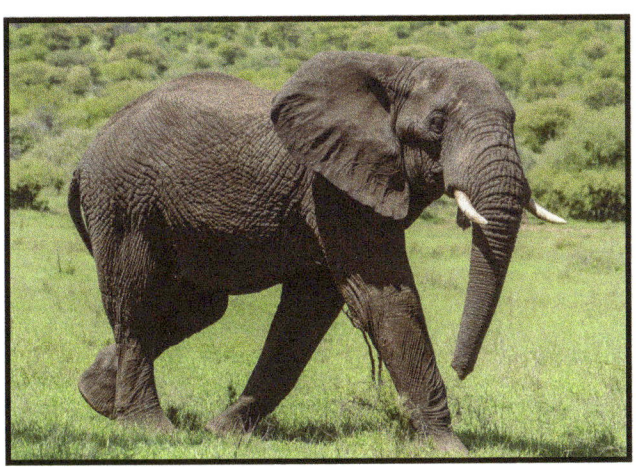

Give the child the parts and tell child to "make them the same". Start by placing the two parts in the correct orientation and close together

Do hand-over-hand to teach the child if necessary

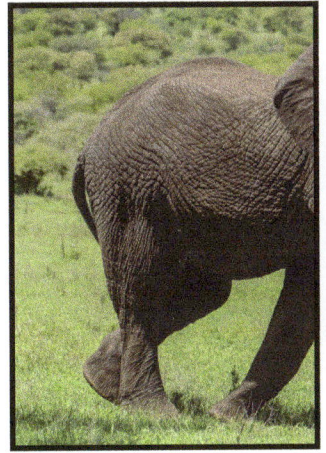
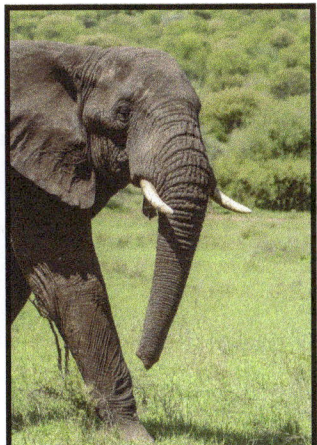

COGNITIVE DEVELOPMENT

⋯→ *Part-Whole Puzzle (continued)*

3 Rotate one side and tell child to "make them the same"

4 Rotate both sides and tell child to "make them the same"

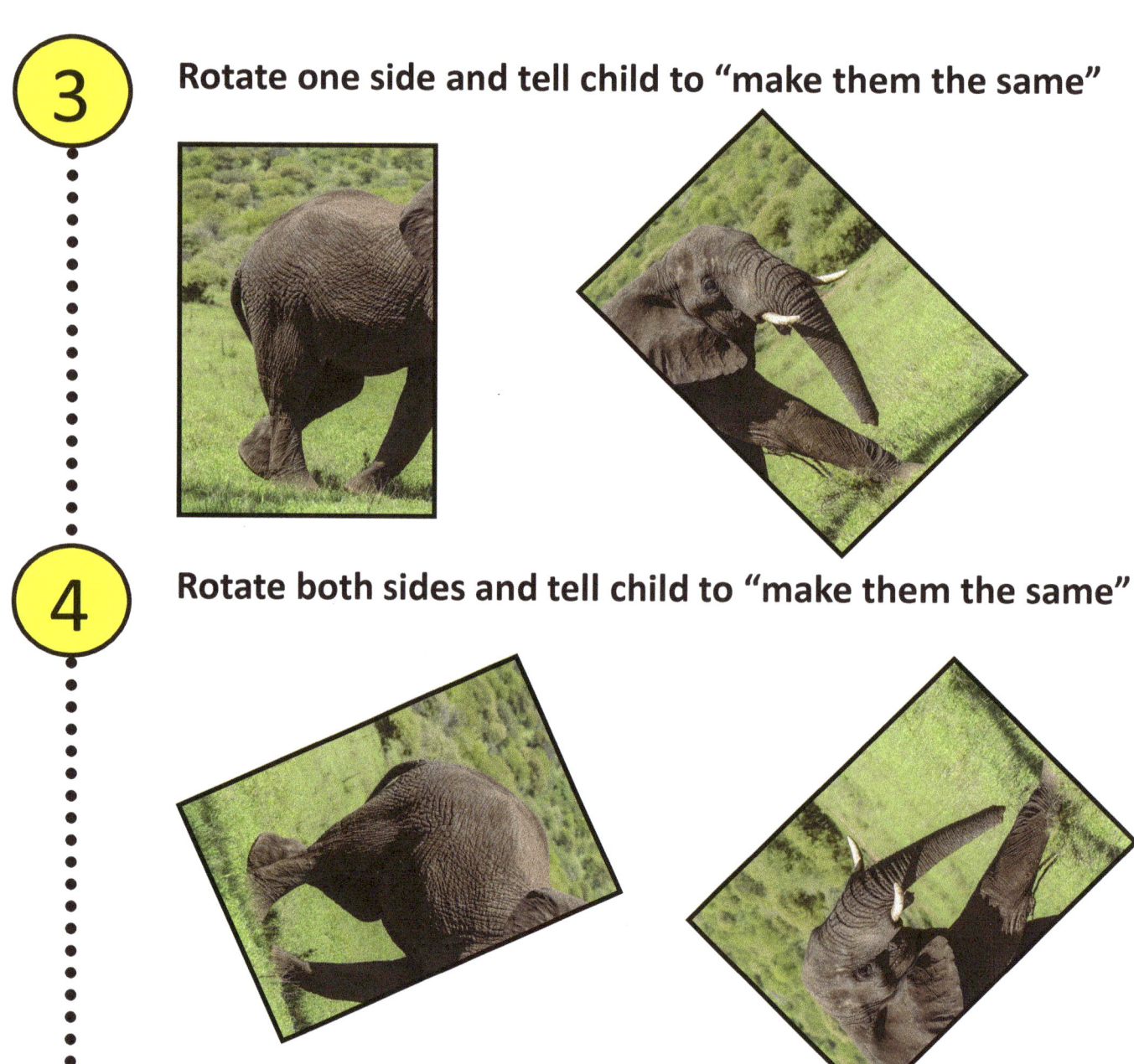

COGNITIVE DEVELOPMENT

···→ *Part-Whole Puzzle (continued)*

 **Remove full picture from table and ask the child to "make the elephant" starting from stage 2**

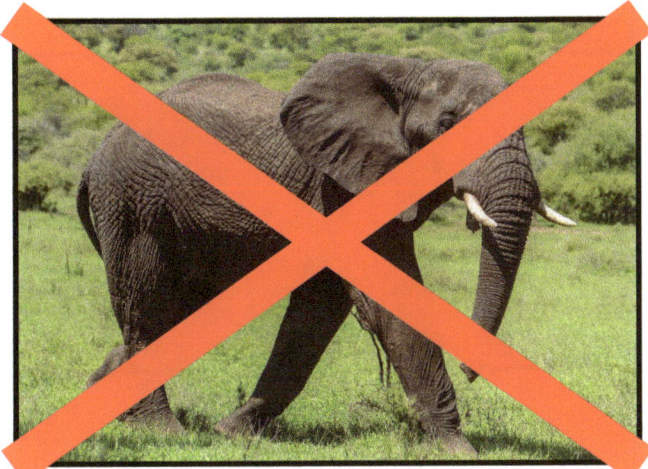

6 **Increase difficulty progressively by increasing the number of parts in the picture**

7 **Start doing jigsaw puzzles**

COGNITIVE DEVELOPMENT

⋯→ *Follow the rule*

- Increase the child's compliance to rules

1 **Parent creates a rule**

Example: Triangle is red, circle is orange, square is green

2 **Child receives an empty task**

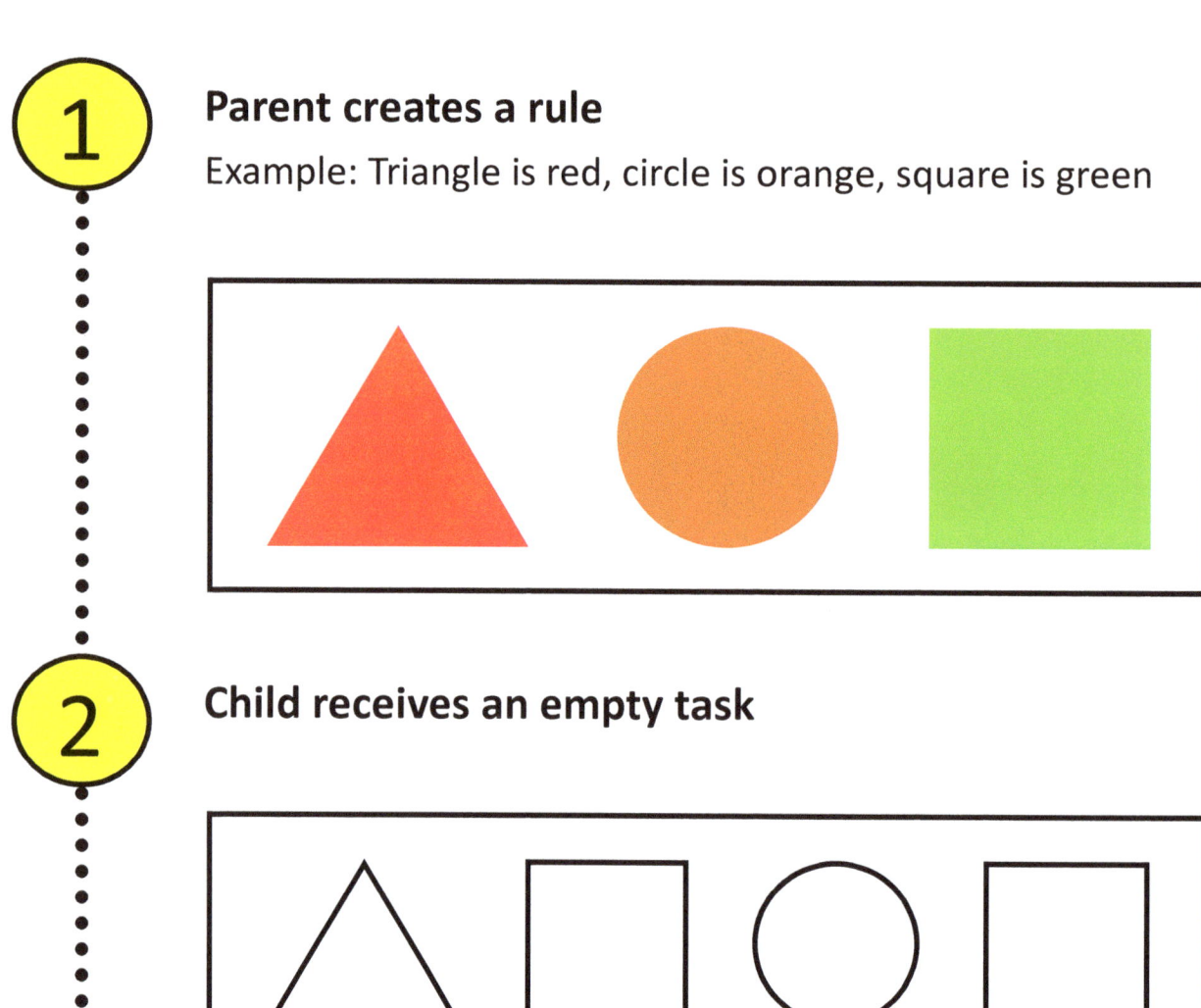

COGNITIVE DEVELOPMENT

⋯→ *Follow the rule (continued)*

 **Child has to color the shapes according to the rule and in order (from left to right)**

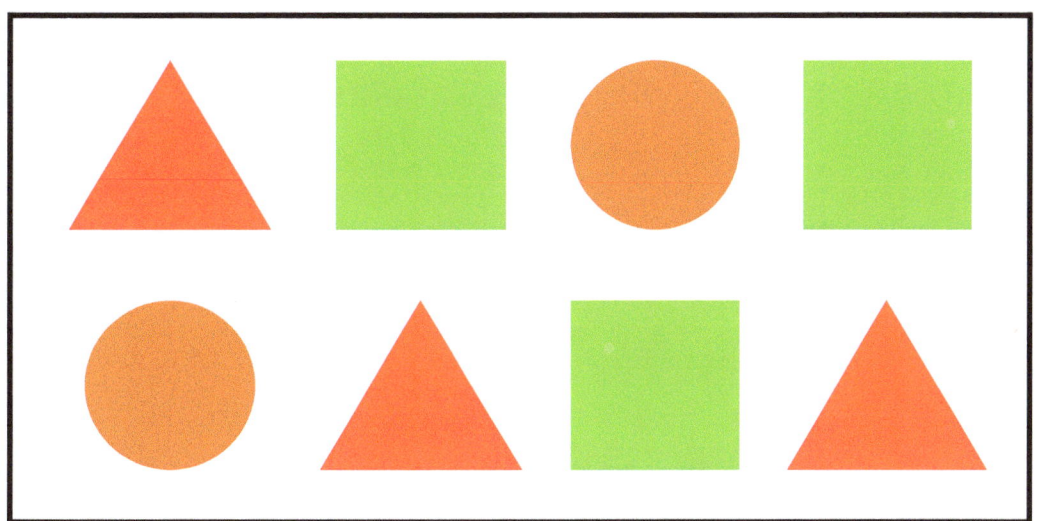

- Initially, parents have to do it together with the child, constantly prompting the child to look back at the rule. Eventually, the goal is for the child to do it independently.

Variations:
- **More rules**
  (E.g., 5 different shapes with 5 different colors)
- **More questions**
  (E.g., child has to color 20 shapes instead of 8 shapes)

LANGUAGE DEVELOPMENT

Children with autism have certain patterns of language and behaviors that are different from typically developing children. EIBI aims to provide intervention that is based on a child with autism's typical learning style and behaviors. These include:

1. repetitive or rigid language

2. narrow interests and exceptional abilities

3. uneven language development and

4. poor non-verbal conversational skills

EIBI targets language development based on four main components:

1. Listening (Receptive language)

2. Speaking (Expressive language)

3. Reading

4. Writing (*in Fine Motor Skills section*)

Receptive vs Expressive Language

Language is also categorized into two important components:

1. **Receptive language**

    - The understanding of language "input"

    - Includes: Words, gestures, interpreting questions and complex grammatical form

2. **Expressive language**

    - The "output" of language: how one expresses wants and needs

    - Includes: Words, grammar rules for phrases, sentences and paragraphs, use of gestures and facial expressions.

All the following have both receptive and expressive components which can be taught in the following order:

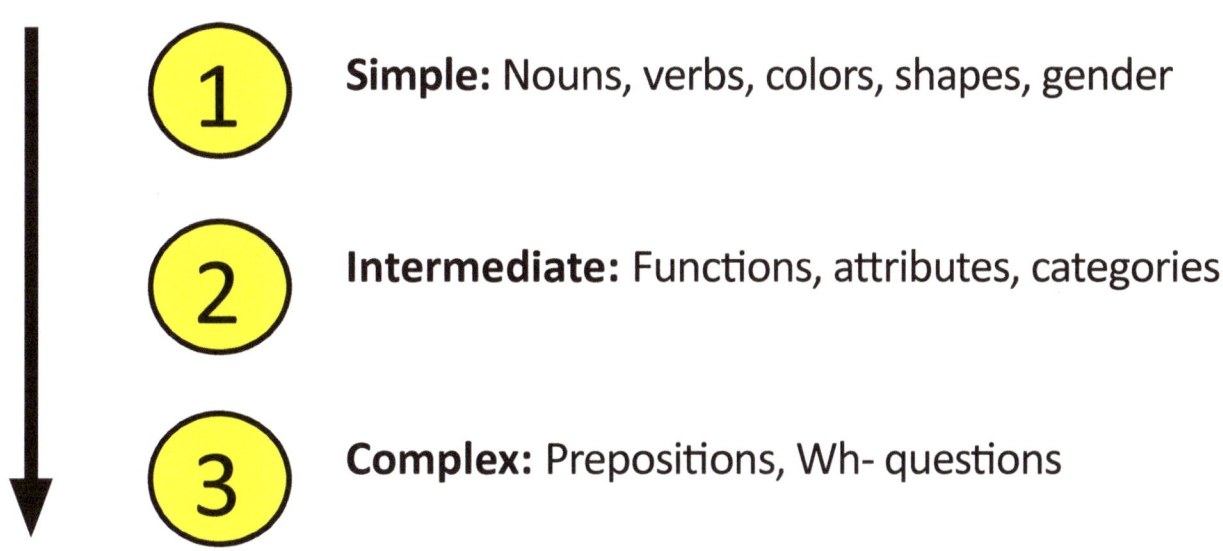

1 **Simple:** Nouns, verbs, colors, shapes, gender

2 **Intermediate:** Functions, attributes, categories

3 **Complex:** Prepositions, Wh- questions

1. Receptive language

⸱⸱⸱→ *Imitation*

- Works on **receptive** aspect of language

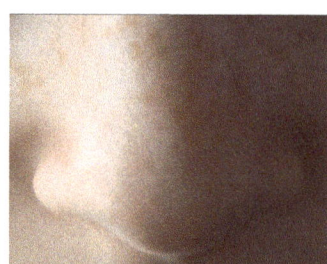

1 **Give child specific instructions with visual cards**

- E.g., "Touch nose"

2 **Do action together with the child**

- Child imitates after you

3 **Slowly wean off doing action**

- Start the action with child, but stop after a while and let the child continue

4 **Verbally say instructions without doing action**

- Child learns to do action by listening to your verbal instructions instead of following your action

1. Receptive language

⋯➤ *Matching*

- This task can be done with different kinds of matching cards.

Examples:

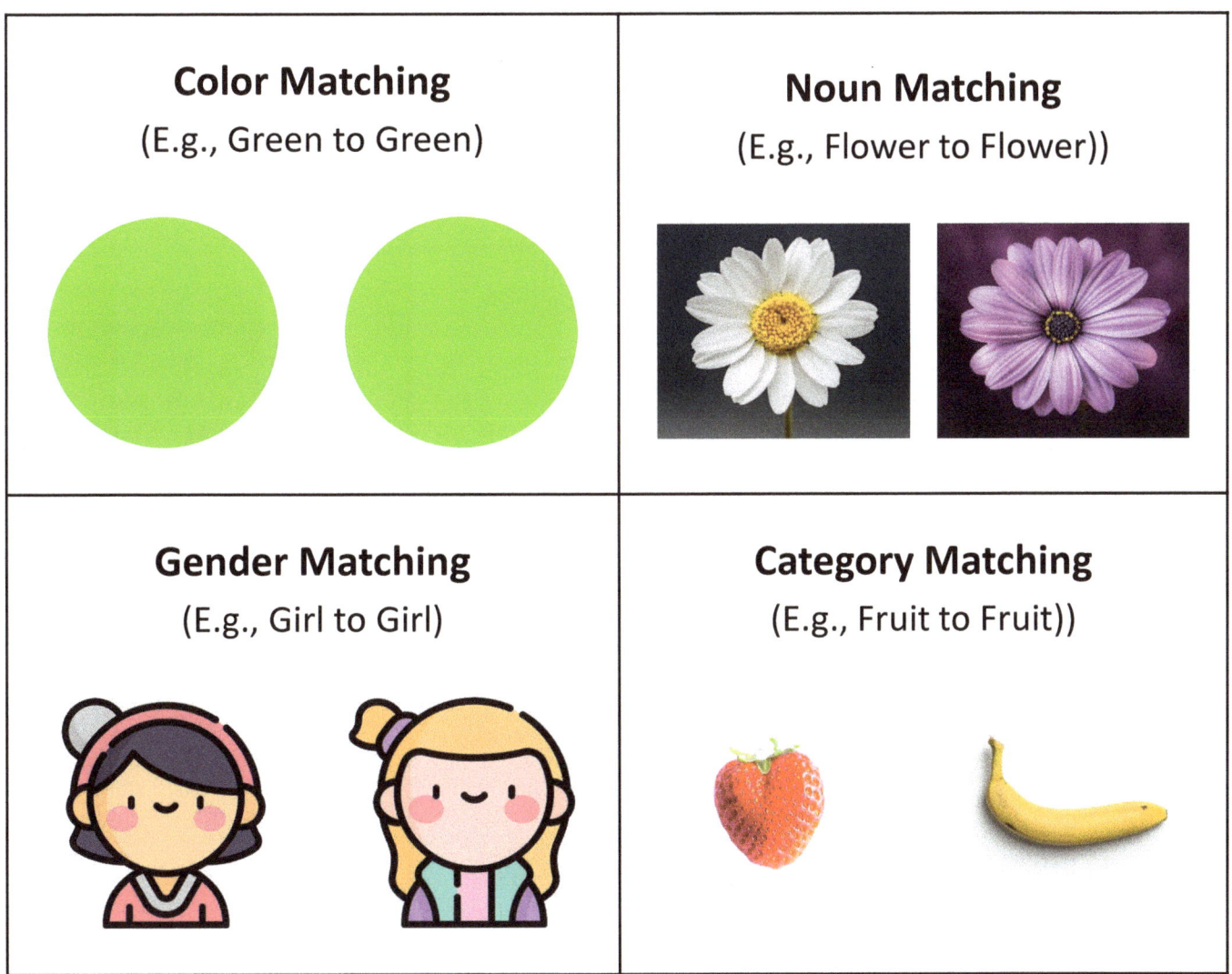

1. Receptive language

⋯→ *Matching (continued)*

- To train child's listening, child has to match cards or pick out cards based on what the parent says.

- Instructions can be given in this order:

1 **"Find same"**

- Parent passes child a card and child has to pick out a card that is the same as the given card.

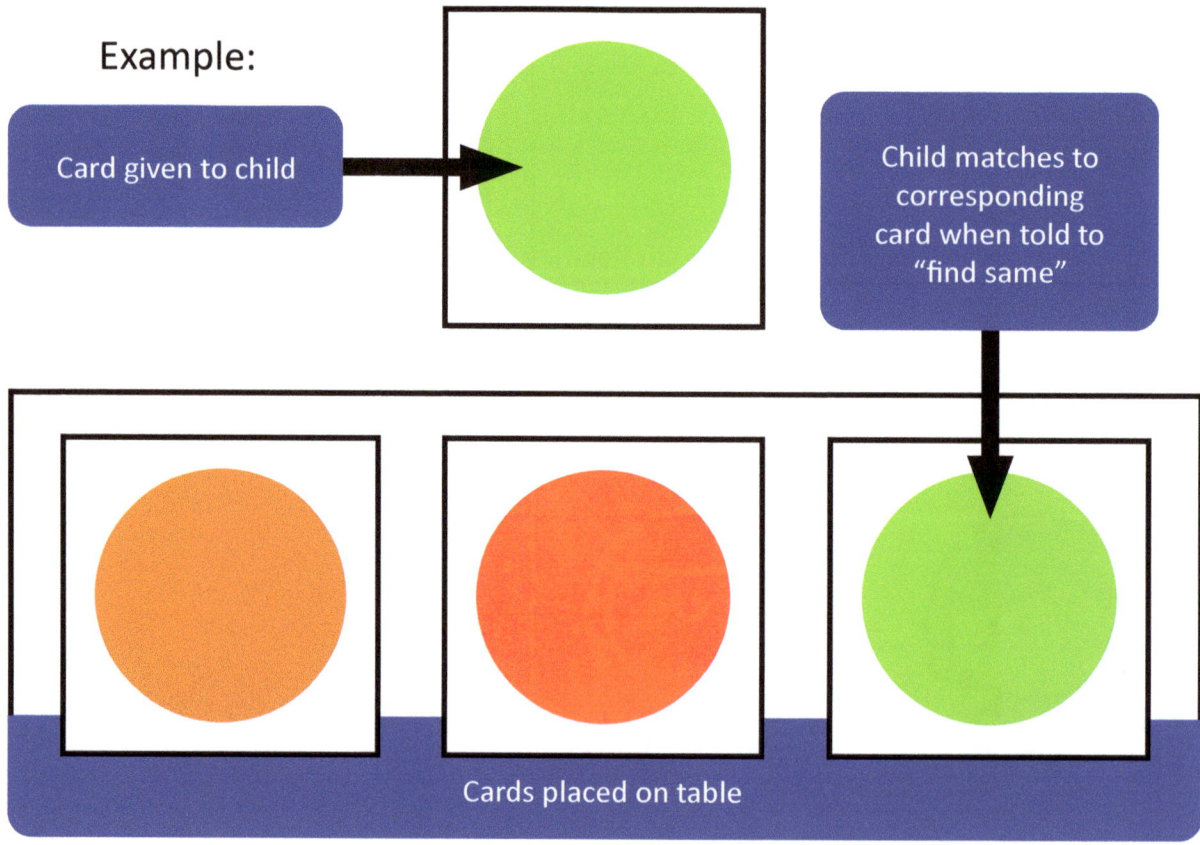

1. Receptive language

···→ *Matching (continued)*

"Give me _____"

- In this stage, child has to listen to what the parent wants and pass the card to the parent

Example:

"Give me red!"

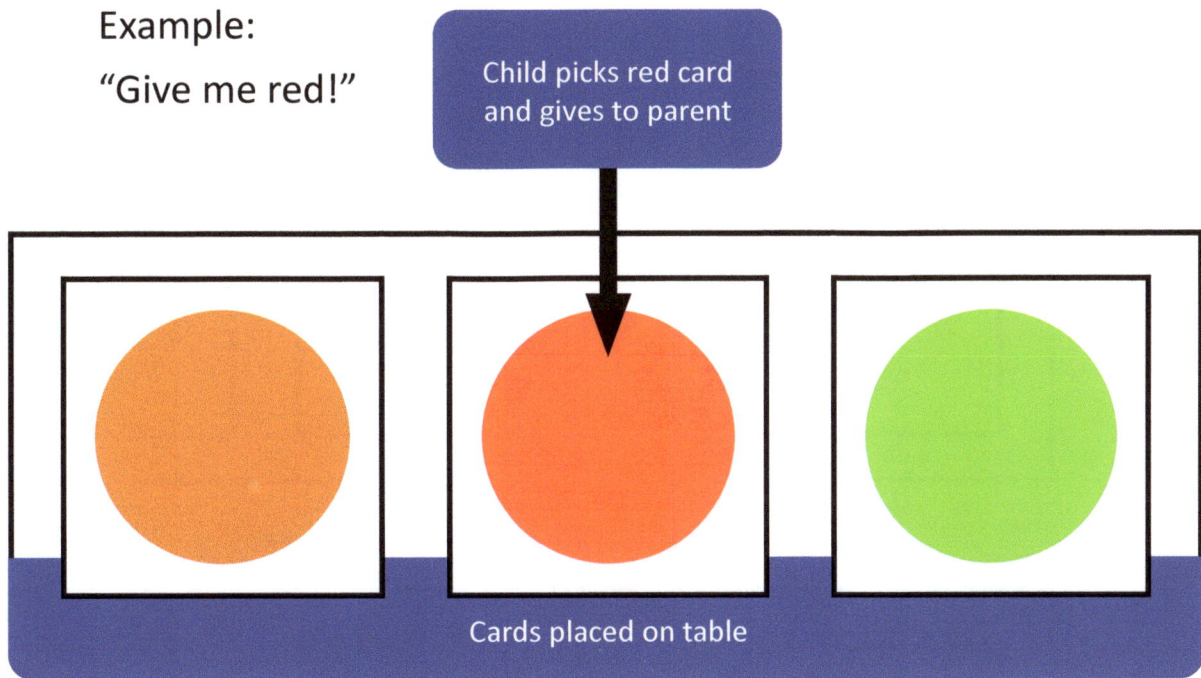

Child picks red card and gives to parent

Cards placed on table

Possible variations

➜ Change action word (E.g., Point to red, Put hand on red)

➜ Increase or decrease number of cards on table

1. Receptive language

···→ *Matching (continued)*

"Show me (Descriptive word)"

- In this stage, parents describe the card instead of naming the card.

Example:

"Show me the color of grass!"

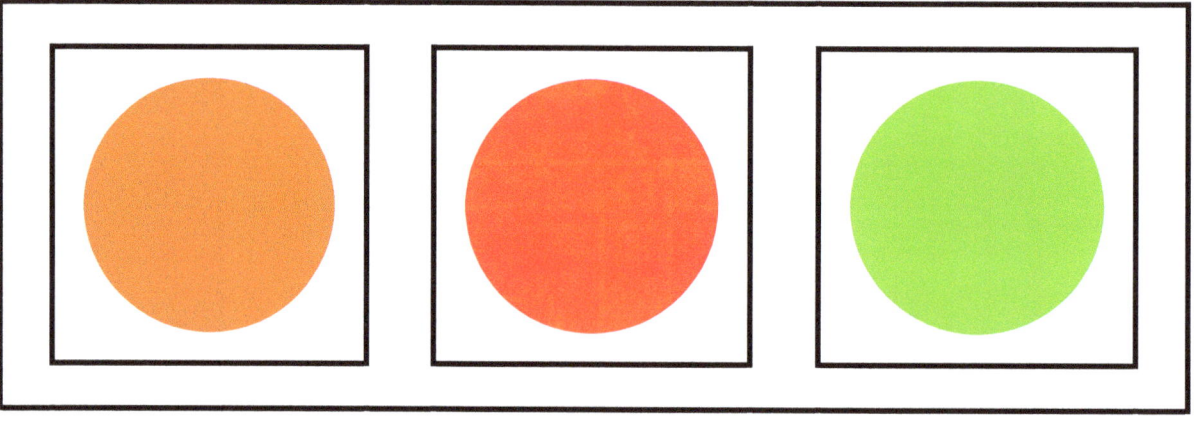

"Show me the something that barks!"

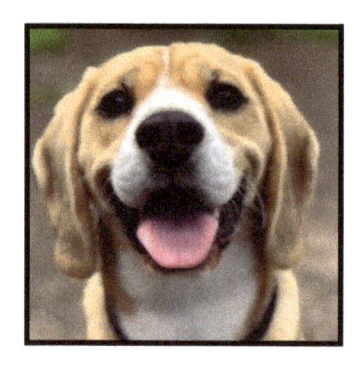 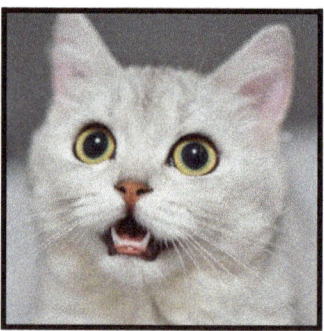 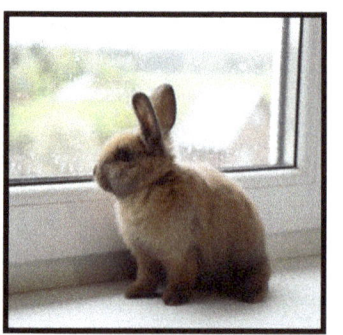

1. Receptive language

┈➤ *Barrier Game (Advanced listening)*

- Works on receptive aspect of language

1   **Each person gets the same items**

2   **Items are hidden behind a barrier**

3   **One person uses words to explain where to place each item**

4   **Remove the barrier to see if everyone managed to create the right figure!**

Variations

➔ Increase or decrease the number of cards on the table

➔ Showing the item mentioned to build vocabulary

2. Expressive language

⋯→ *Picture Exchange Communication System (PECS)*

- To teach **functional** communication skills with an initial focus on **spontaneous communication**.

- Verbal prompts are **not used** during the early phases, thus building immediate initiation and avoiding prompt dependency.

Simplified PECS board

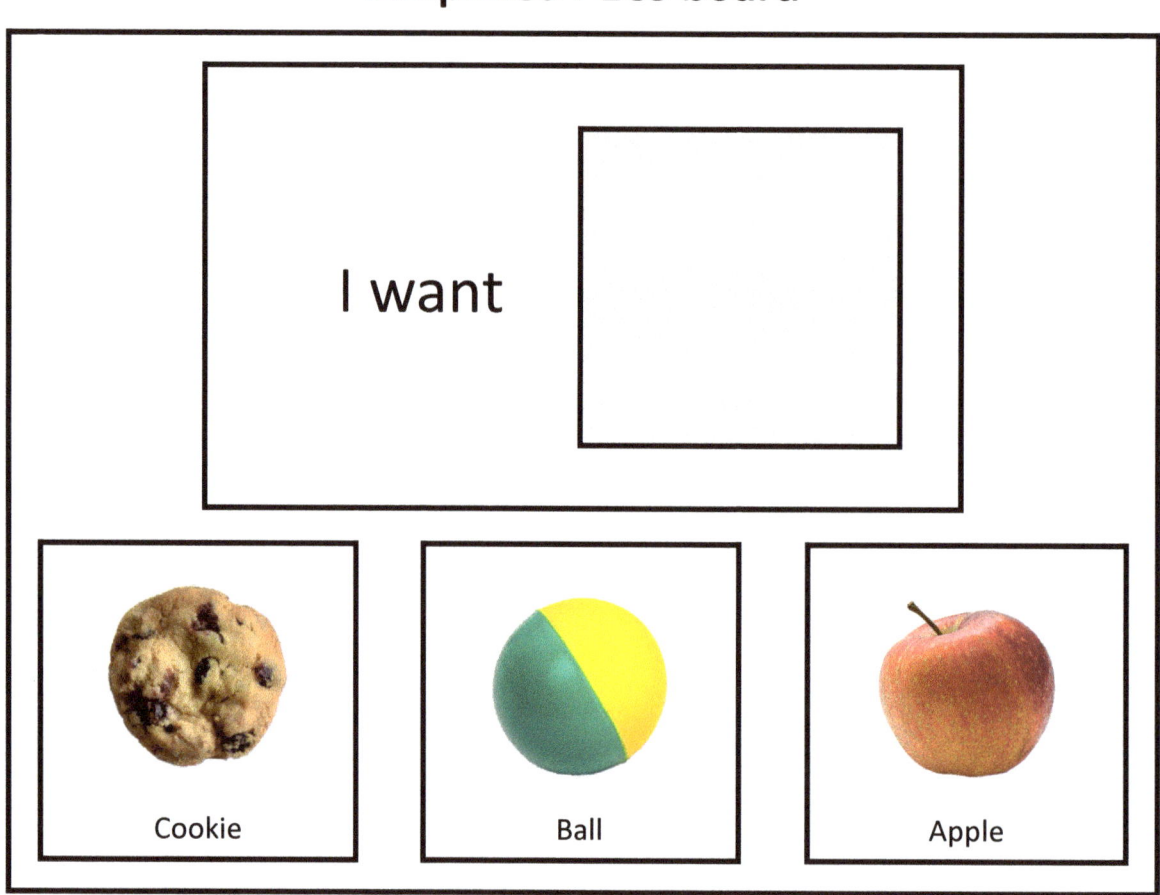

2. Expressive language

⋯→ *PECS (continued)*

HOW CAN I USE PECS?

Create a PECS board

- Start simple, with a few items the child constantly requests.
- Cards should include pictures of the items.

Example:

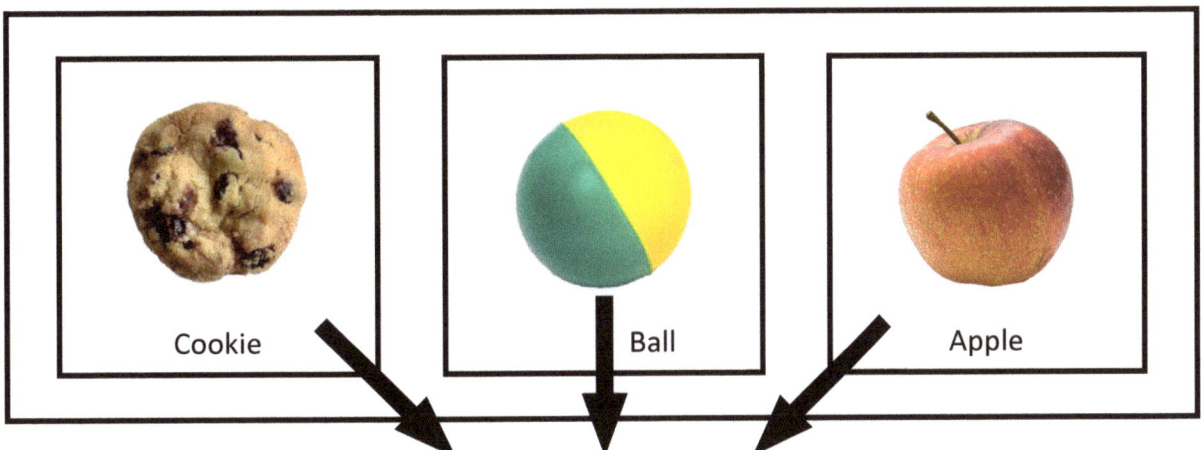

| Cookie | Ball | Apple |

Each item card is individually pasted on a board using velcro or bluetack. **Cards must be able to be detached from the board!**

Place it in a place the child can easily access

- Within child's reach (not placed too high)
- Child must be able to see it (not placed inside a drawer)
- Good places include the wall in the living room

⋯→ *PECS (continued)*

3 Child requests items by taking the corresponding card out from the board and passing it to the parent

4 Once child passes parent the card, parent verbalizes for them (E.g.,"John wants milk!") and encourages child to verbalize as well.

> *Do NOT force if child doesn't verbalize.

5 Parent passes to child the item requested

6 Card is then placed back onto the PECS board for future use

7 Continue to engage in PECS progression to help child progress in language & communication (next section)

···→ *PECS (continued)*

PECS Progression

Progression in PECS helps child progress and learn new phrases and sentences for communication. The following acts as a guideline for PECS progression.

How to communicate (Teaching phase)

- To guide the child on how to use PECS, parents can create a simple board with only 2-3 item cards on it.

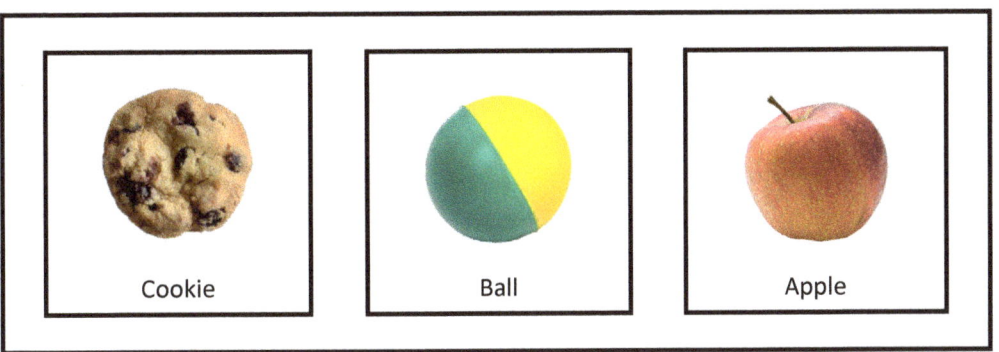

- Ideally, 2 adults are needed for teaching phase: Adult 1 acts as the receiver, while Adult 2 acts as the prompter.

- Prompter uses hand-over-hand with the child to take out an item card from the PECS board and passes it to the receiver together with the child.

- The adult receiving the card then gives the child the item on the card.

- This process must be done repeatedly and consistently for the child to learn.

- Eventually, prompter weans off, and child learns how to communicate with PECS.

⸱⸱⸱→ *PECS (continued)*

2 **Distance**

- Once child is familiar with communicating using PECS, parents can move farther away from the child and get the child to walk to them to give the card.

3 **Discrimination between symbols**

- At this stage, more item cards can be added...

- Progressively introduce more item cards.

- Item cards should be cards of items that child frequently requests (e.g., specific toy, specific food or places).

- Child then learns to discriminate between the different symbols.

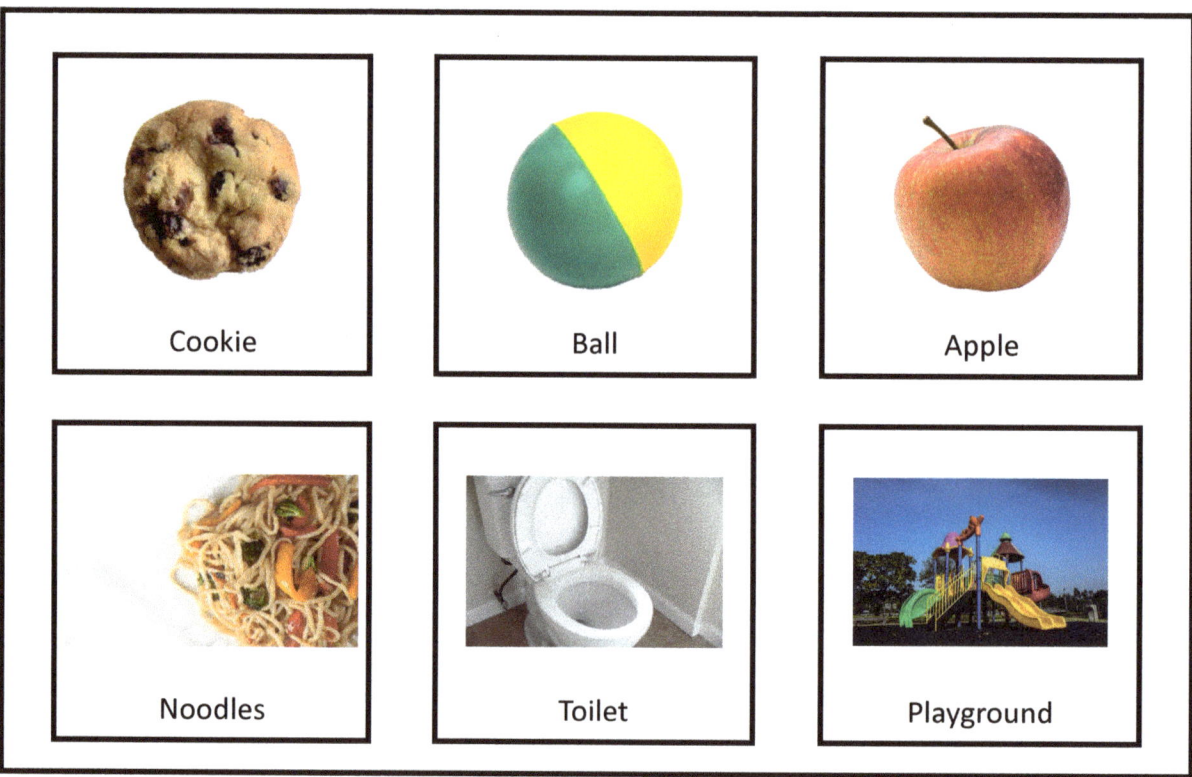

Cookie	Ball	Apple
Noodles	Toilet	Playground

⋯→ *PECS (continued)*

Using phrases

- At this stage, the child can start learning to use phrases.

- The PECS board can be updated to include a **communication strip** like shown below.

- To request, child has to stick the item card on the communication strip, and then pass the entire strip to the adult.

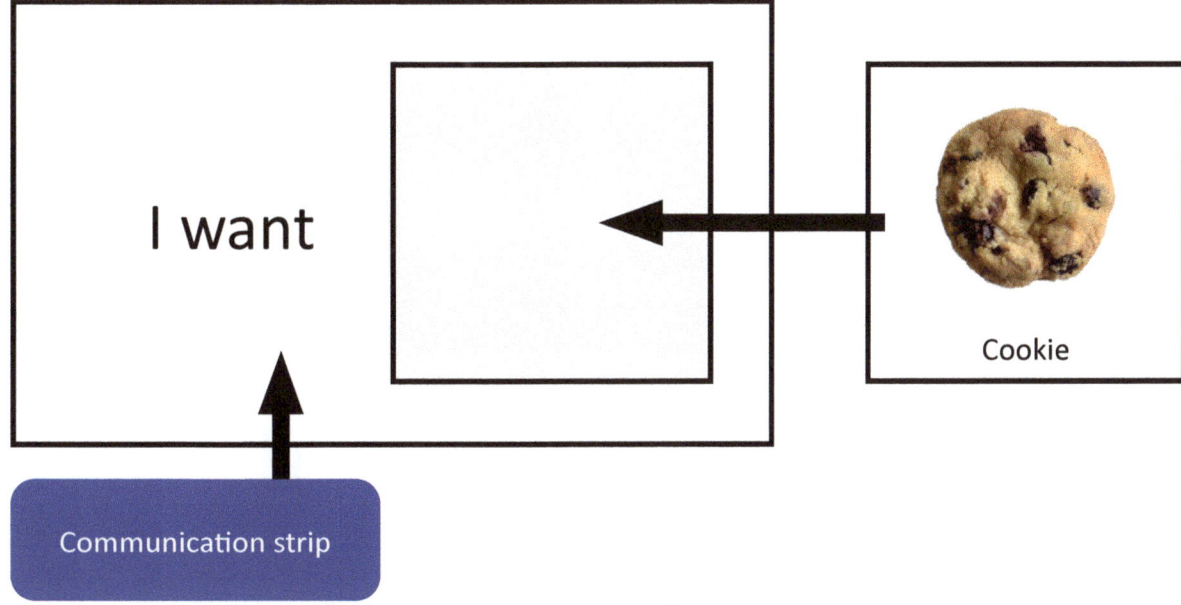

- The adult can try getting the child to verbally say the phrase after child passes over the communication strip (e.g., getting child to repeat after adult). **However, do not force the child to verbally request. Item should still be given to the child as long as the communication strip is passed to the adult (even with no words spoken).**

- If the child attempts to verbalize but did not articulate clearly, do NOT correct but instead encourage with "Wow! Good try!"

⋯→ *PECS (continued)*

 **Using phrases (continued)**

- Child can also learn simple greeting phrases as follows:

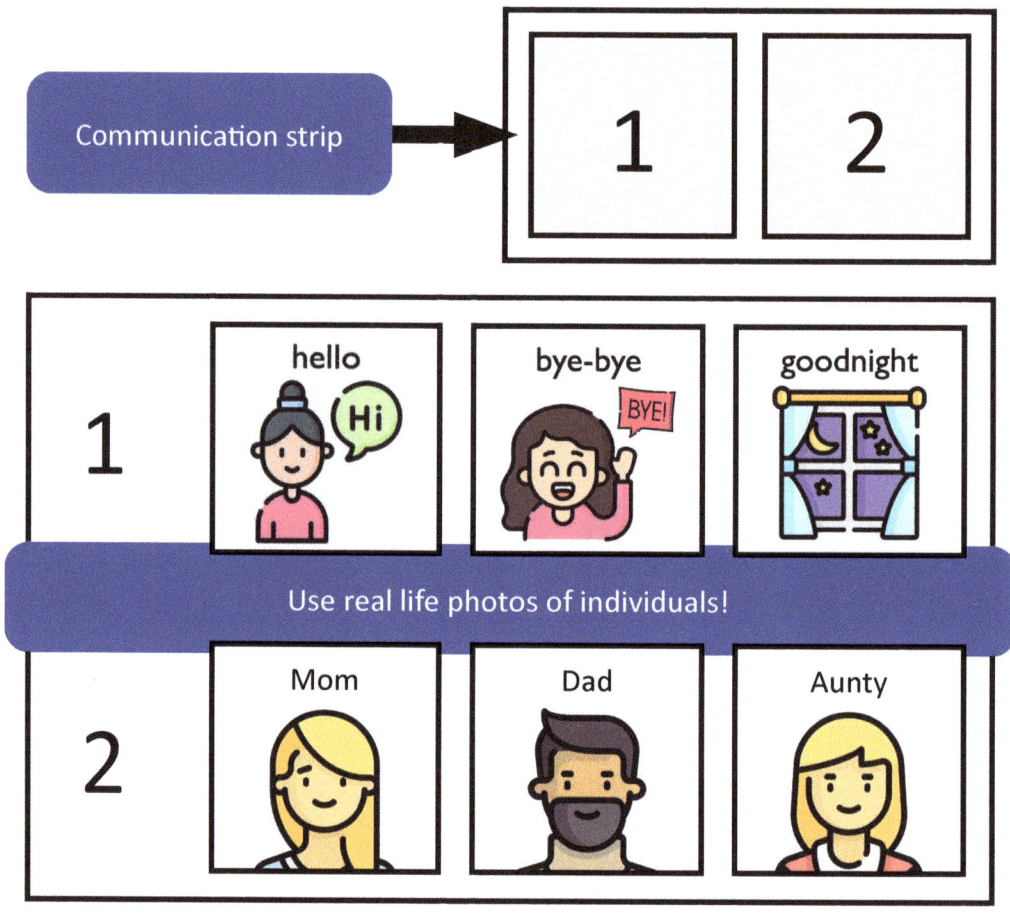

- Child then pick the appropriate cards to paste on the communication strip and pass it to the respective individual.

Example:

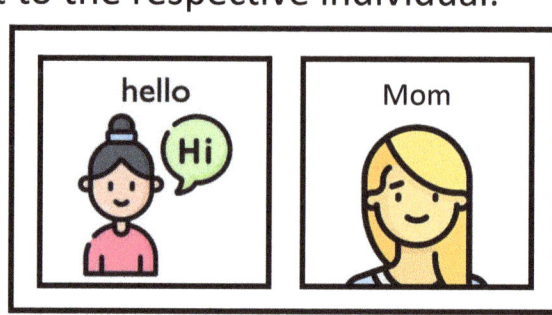

⋯→ *PECS (continued)*

Sentence building

- Child can then start to build sentences in the following progression:

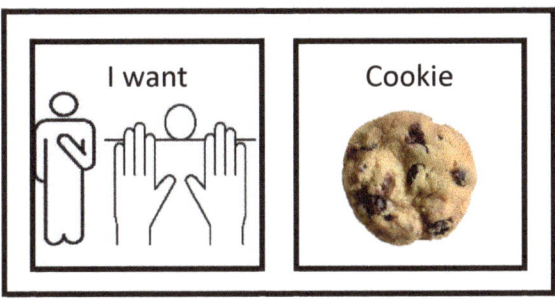

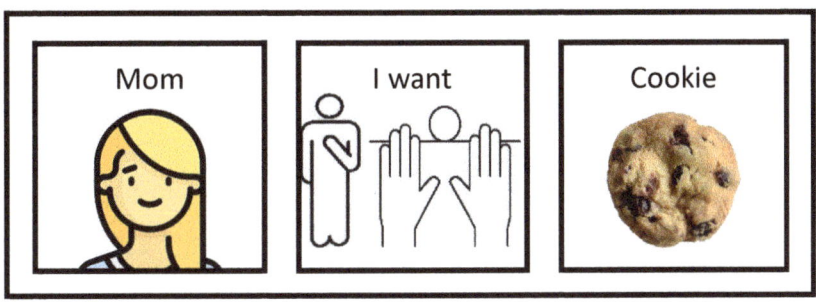

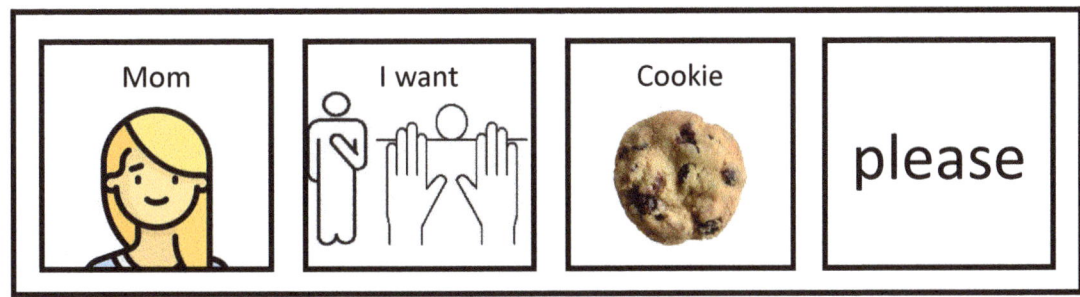

Consistency is key!

3. Reading

⋯→ *Letter & Phonic Recognition*

- For the child to learn how to read words, the child must first recognize letters and associate the letter to its phonic.

- This can be done in the following stages:

① **Matching letter to letter (uppercase)**
- Ask child to "find same" or "find A"

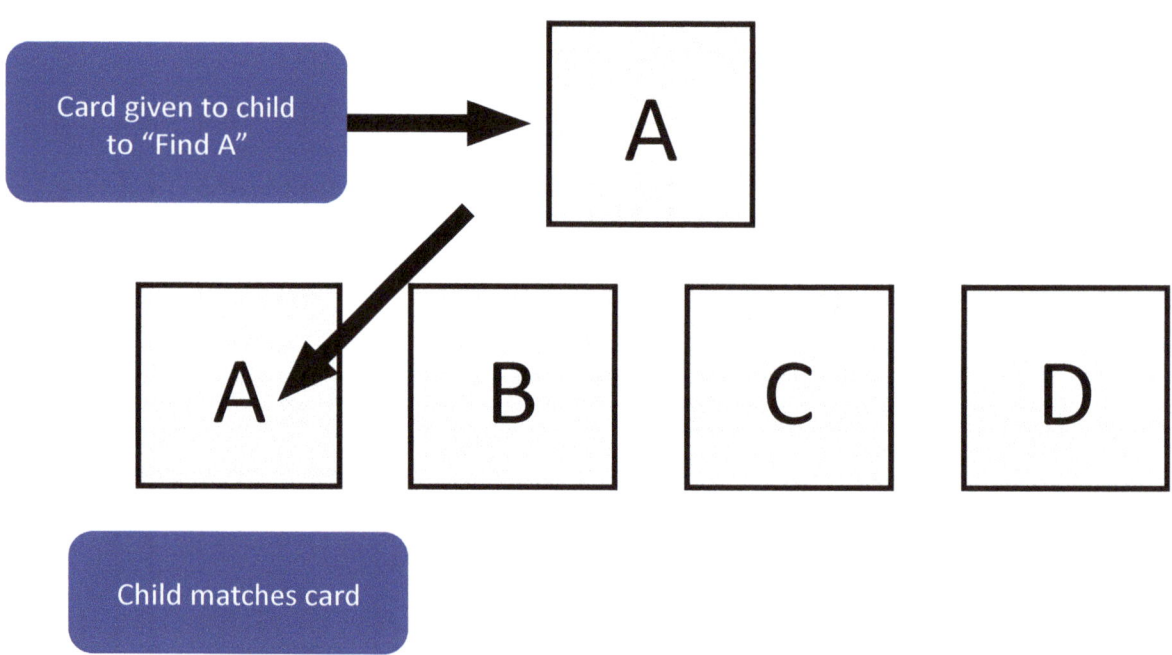

···→ *Letter & Phonic Recognition (continued)*

2 **Matching letter to letter (lowercase)**

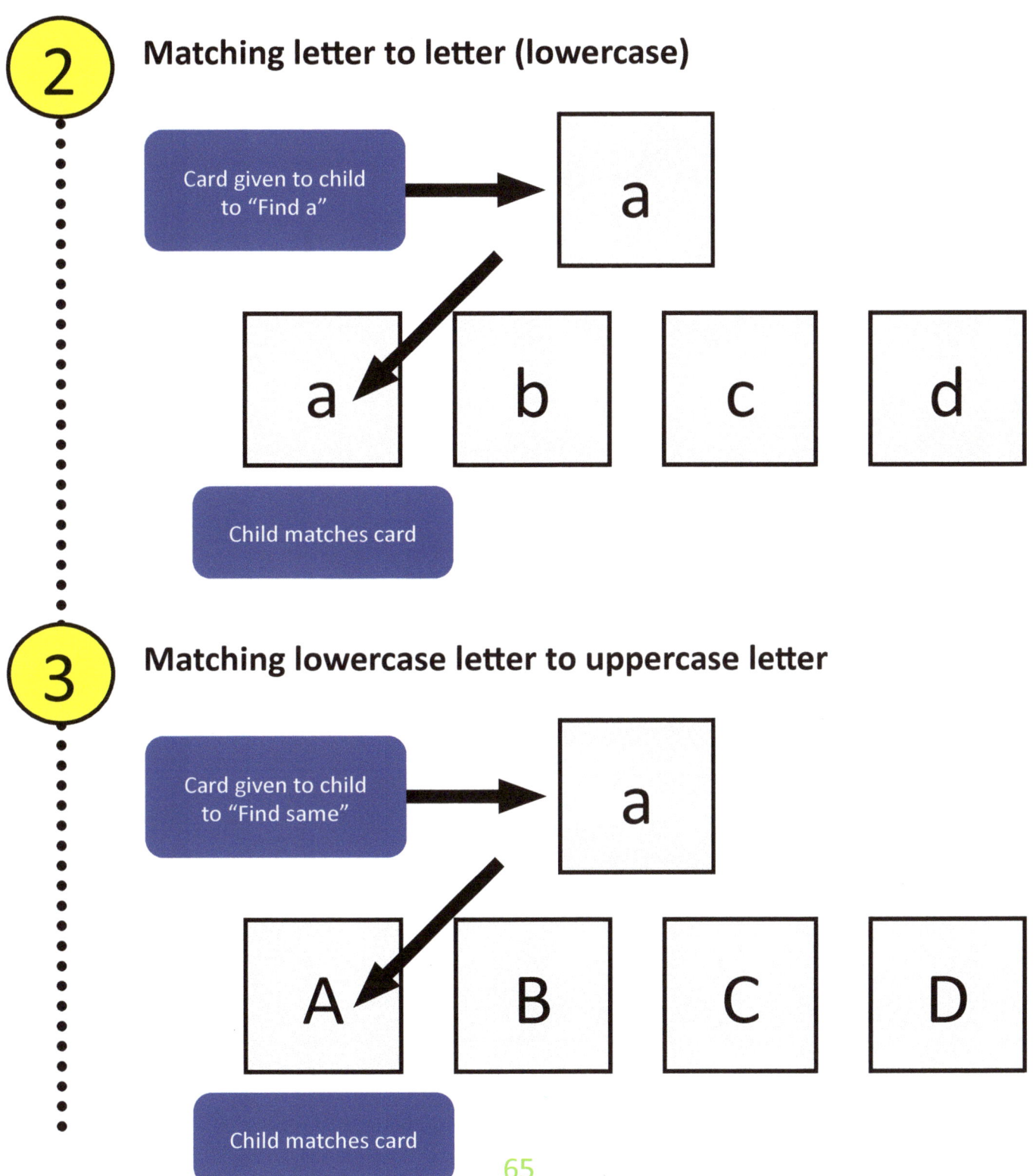

3 **Matching lowercase letter to uppercase letter**

⇢ *Letter & Phonic Recognition (continued)*

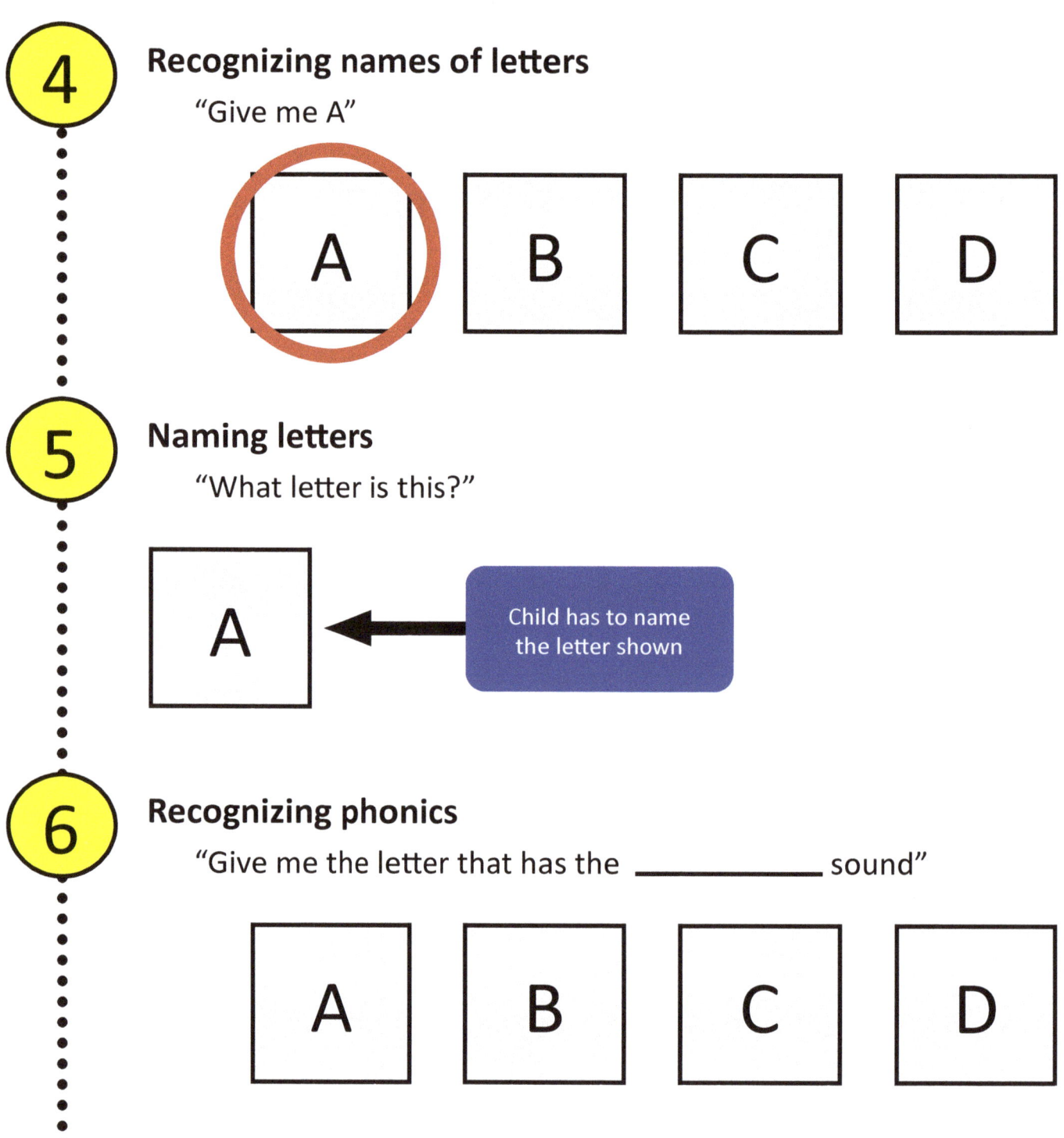

4 **Recognizing names of letters**

"Give me A"

A | B | C | D

5 **Naming letters**

"What letter is this?"

A ← Child has to name the letter shown

6 **Recognizing phonics**

"Give me the letter that has the _____ sound"

A | B | C | D

⤏ *Letter & Phonic Recognition (continued)*

 **Phonic production**

"What is the sound of this letter?"

A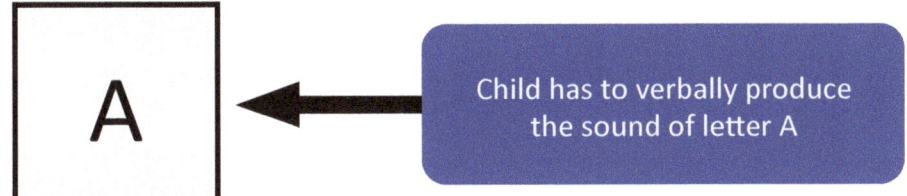

Child has to verbally produce the sound of letter A

 **Phonics blending**

- Once the child knows all the phonics for the individual letters, the child can proceed to learn phonics blending for 2-letter blends.

- Here is a list of blends parents can start with:

ch	sh	th	wh	ar	ay
oo	ow	ee	ey	er	ir
ur	oy	oi	ou	aw	ew

3. Reading

⋯→ *Sight Words*

- Once the child learns phonics, he is ready to learn sight words.

HOW CAN I TEACH SIGHT WORDS?

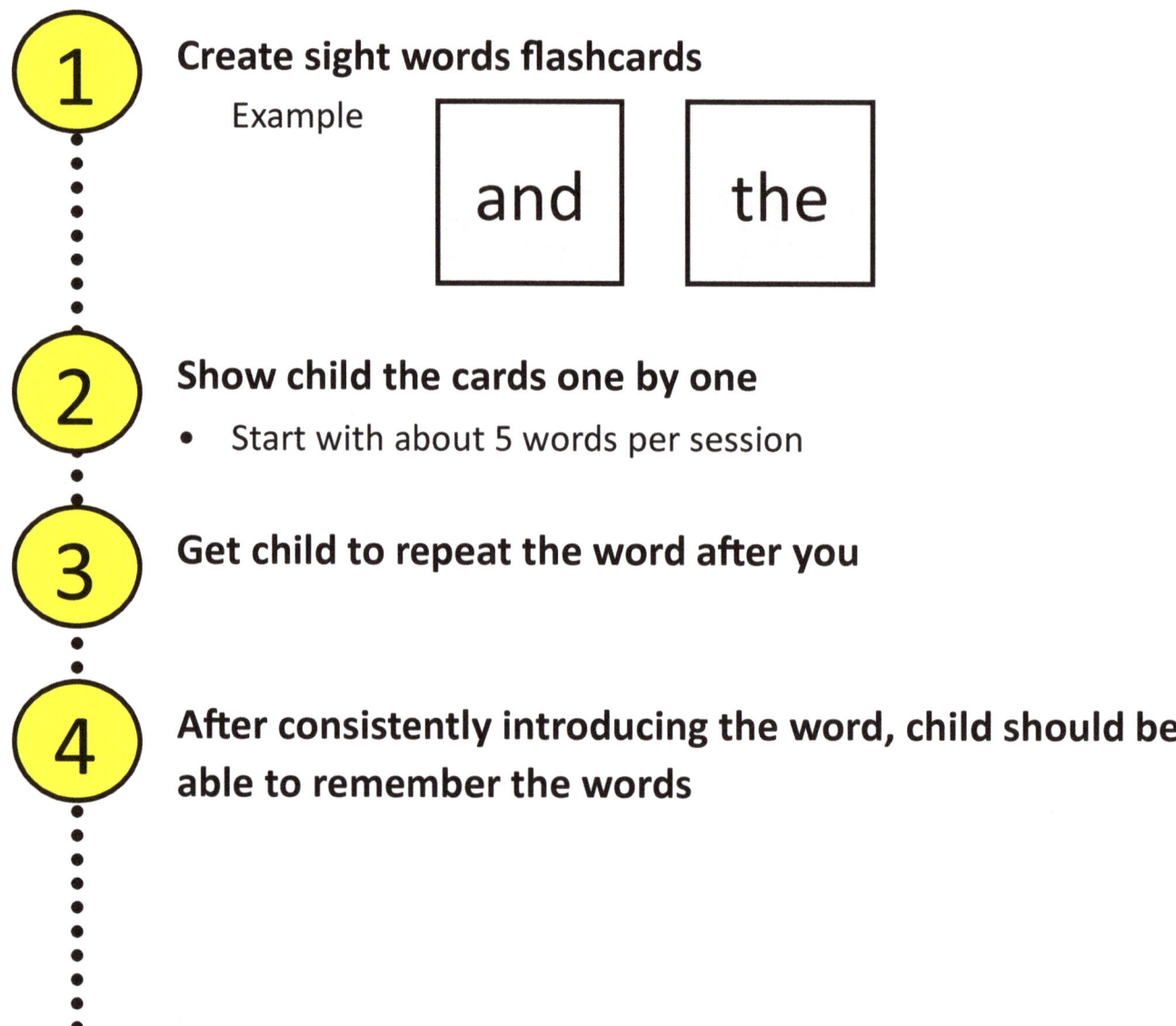

1   **Create sight words flashcards**

Example

| and | the |

2   **Show child the cards one by one**

- Start with about 5 words per session

3   **Get child to repeat the word after you**

4   **After consistently introducing the word, child should be able to remember the words**

┄→ *Sight Words (continued)*

LIST OF SIGHT WORDS (DOLCH'S SIGHT WORDS)

- Below are lists of high-frequency words that can be taught to the child based on age and ability.

Preschool Sight Words

the	to	and	a
I	you	it	in
said	for	up	look
is	go	we	little
down	can	see	not
one	my	me	big
come	blue	red	where
jump	away	here	help
make	yellow	two	play
run	find	three	funny

Kindergarten Sight Words

he	was	that	she
on	they	but	at
with	all	there	out
be	have	am	do
did	what	so	get
like	this	will	yes
went	are	now	no
came	ride	into	good
want	too	pretty	four
saw	well	ran	brown
eat	who	new	must
black	white	soon	our
ate	say	under	please

Primary 1 sight words

of	his	had	him
her	some	as	then
could	when	where	them
ask	an	over	just
from	any	how	know
put	take	every	old
by	after	think	let
going	walk	again	may
stop	fly	round	give
once	open	has	live

Primary 2 sight words

would	very	your	its
around	don't	right	green
their	call	sleep	five
wash	or	before	been
off	cold	tell	work
first	does	goes	write
always	made	gave	us
buy	those	use	fast
pull	both	sit	which
read	why	found	because
best	upon	these	sing

Primary 3 sight words

if	long	about	got
six	never	seven	eight
today	myself	much	keep
try	start	ten	bring
drink	only	better	hold
warm	full	done	light
pick	hurt	cut	kind
fall	carry	small	own
show	hot	far	draw
clean	grow	together	shall

Chapter 4

FUNCTIONAL SKILLS TRAINING

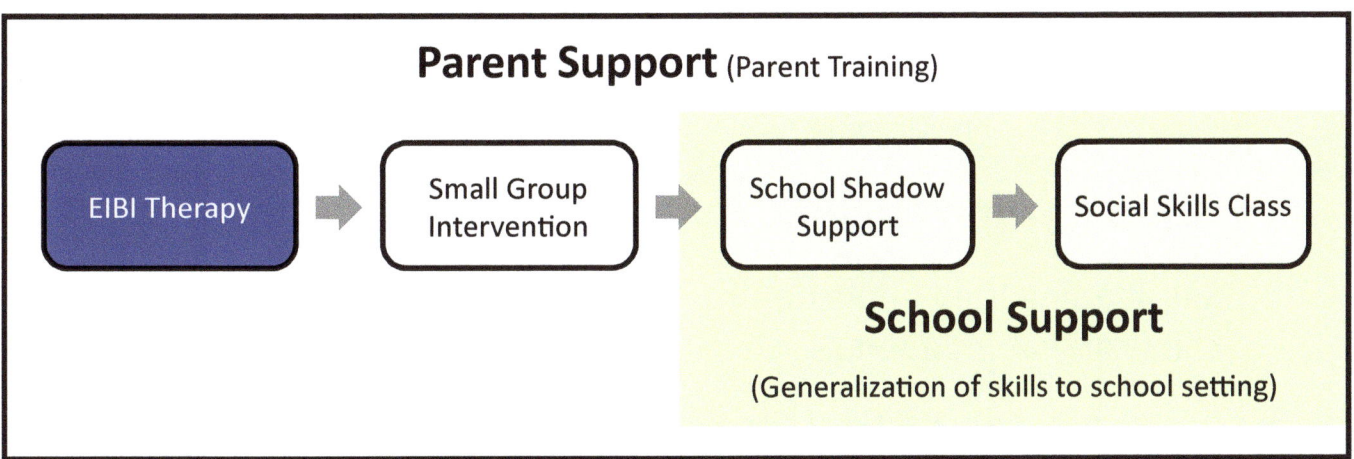

While children go through EIBI therapy, parents can also train them in functional skills such as feeding and toileting. This chapter explains the process for training these skills.

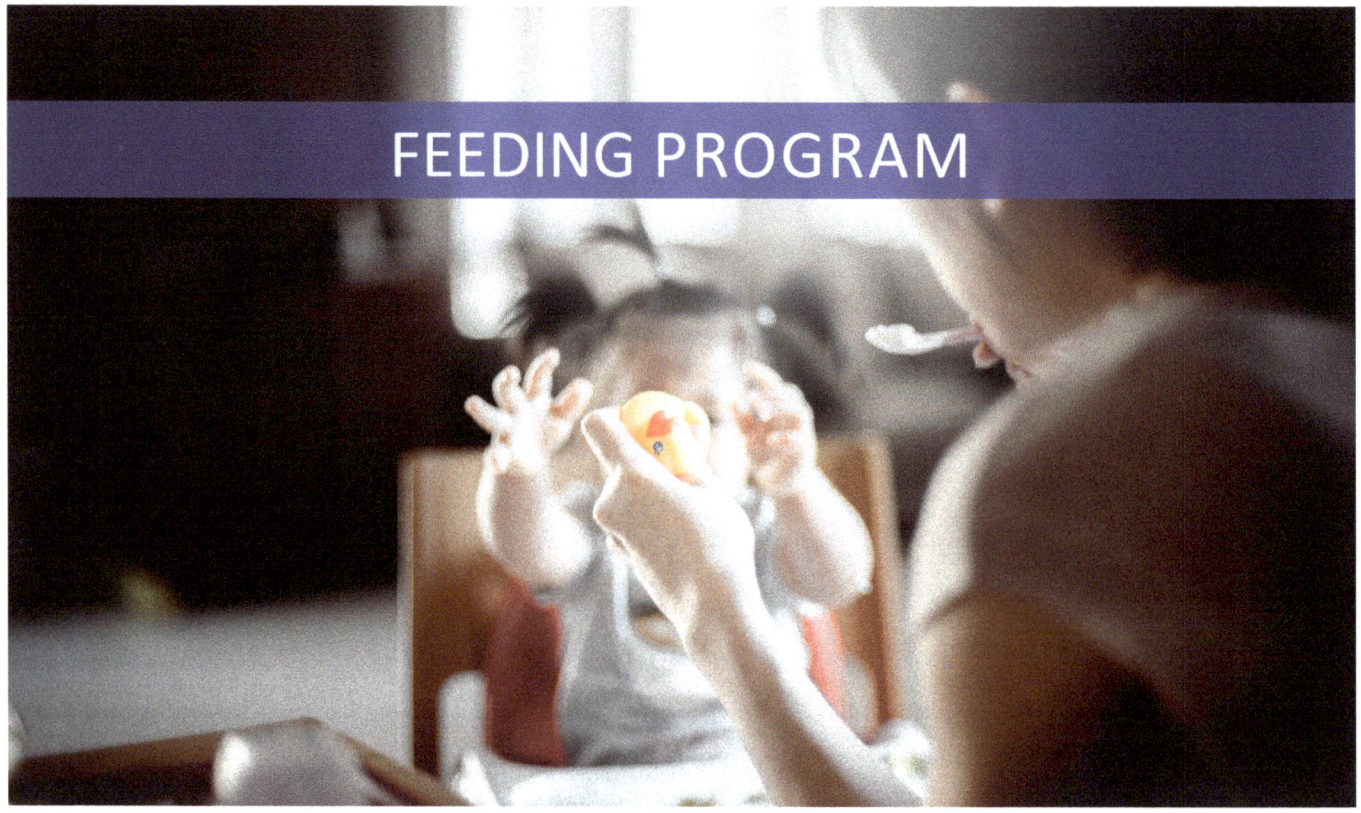

···→ *What is self-feeding?*

- Self-feeding is an important daily living skill to acquire, meaning a child can eat independently without assistance.

- It is also a self-care skill that promotes the child's personal, social and motor development.

FEEDING PROGRAM

⋯→ *Assessing a child's readiness*

- Before starting the feeding program, it is first necessary to determine if the child is ready for it.

- Parents can use the checklist below to assess the child's readiness:

Feeding Program Readiness Checklist

❑ Child is able to sit independently and in a stable position

❑ Child possesses fine motor skills that enables them to hold cutleries

❑ Most of the child's teeth have erupted

❑ Child is able to sustain attention on feeding task

❑ Child is able to comprehend verbal or non-verbal demands from caregivers

❑ Child is able to recognize signs of hunger and is aware of the need to consume food when hungry

❑ Child is mostly compliant during previous feeding sessions

⋯→ *Preparation*

Gathering information

Be aware of:

→ Child's feeding habits

→ Child's dietary restrictions

→ Other common reactions or behaviors

Preparing materials

→ Feeding token economy (see next page)

→ Exclusive reinforcer/reward that a child is likely to value and which a child can only receive exclusively during the course of the feeding program

→ Plastic bowl and plastic cutleries that are safe for the child's use

→ Tissue or wet wipes for the child to use in case of spilled food or messes

⋯→ *Preparation (continued)*

Preparing materials (continued)

Example of Token Economy for Feeding

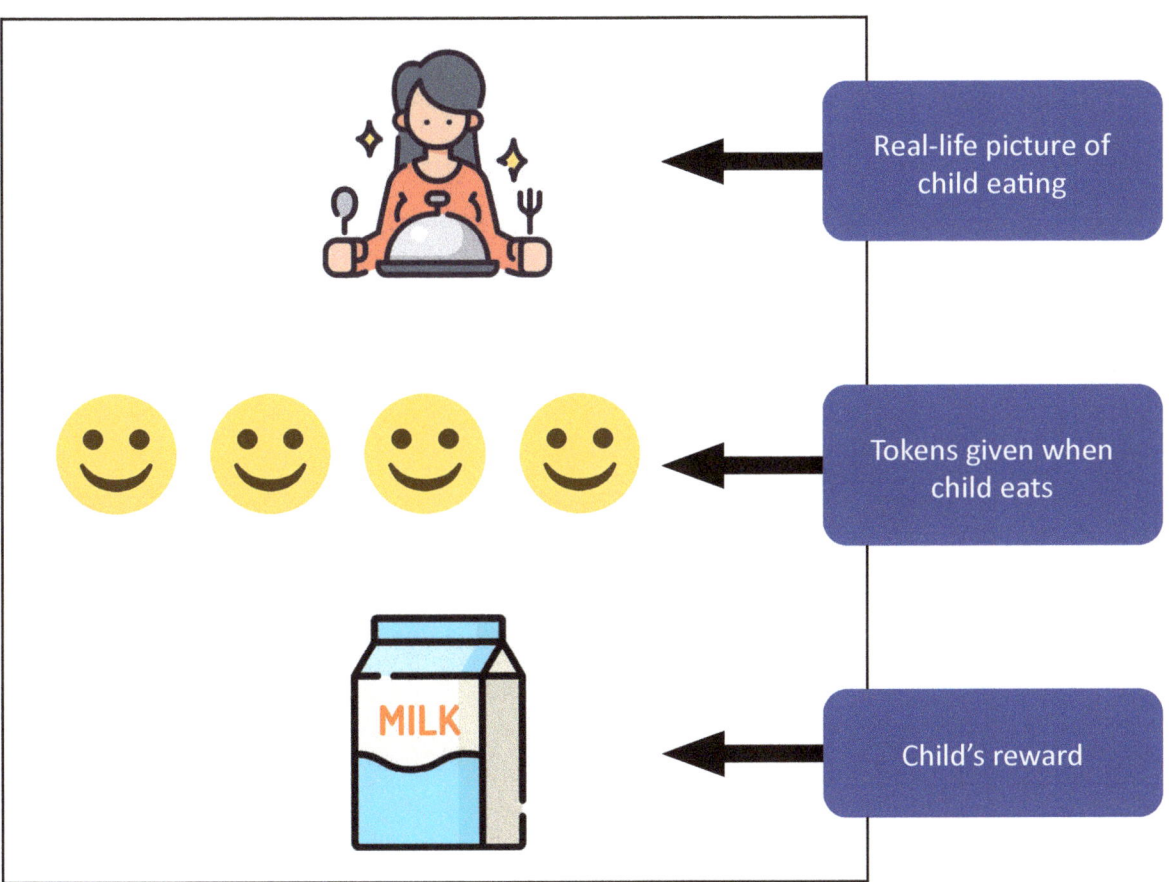

Reward should be *effective* and *exclusive*

➔ *Effective reward:* Reward selected for the feeding program should be one that the child is sufficiently motivated to attain

➔ *Exclusive reward:* Child is only able to obtain this reward during the feeding program, not at any other time of the day!

⇢ *Preparation (continued)*

Preparation of environment

→ Toys, electronic devices, and other distractions should be placed out of reach and out of sight from the child.

→ Furniture (table, chair) should be appropriate based on the size of the child to ensure a comfortable feeding position.

→ Table should only have (1) token economy, (2) tissue, (3) bowl of food. Remove everything else. Reward is to be kept out of sight until enough tokens are earned.

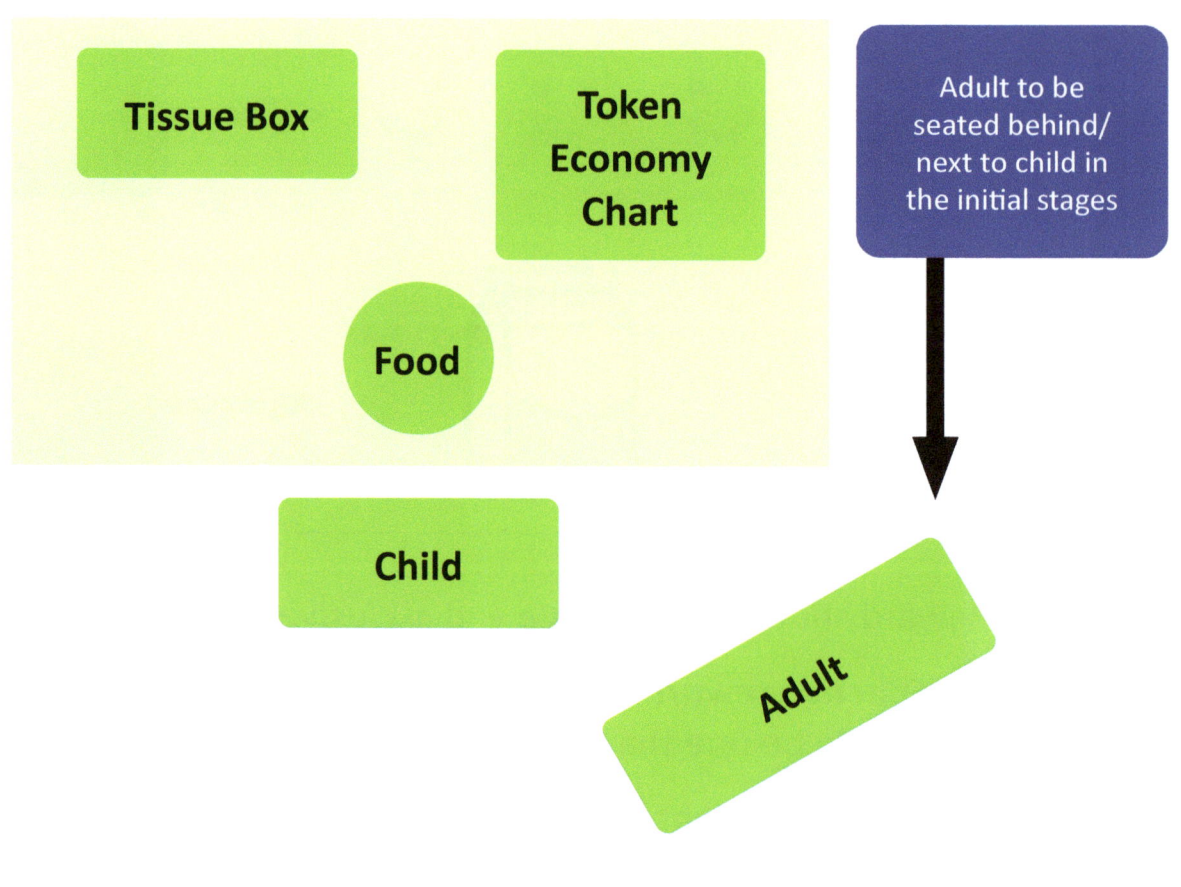

⋯→ *Preparation (continued)*

Schedule meal times

→ Schedule 3 mealtimes a day.

→ Include these mealtimes in the child's daily schedule so the child is aware.

→ Pictures of food can also be shown to the child in advance so the child is prepared.

→ Duration of each mealtime is based on the average time the child takes to complete a meal.

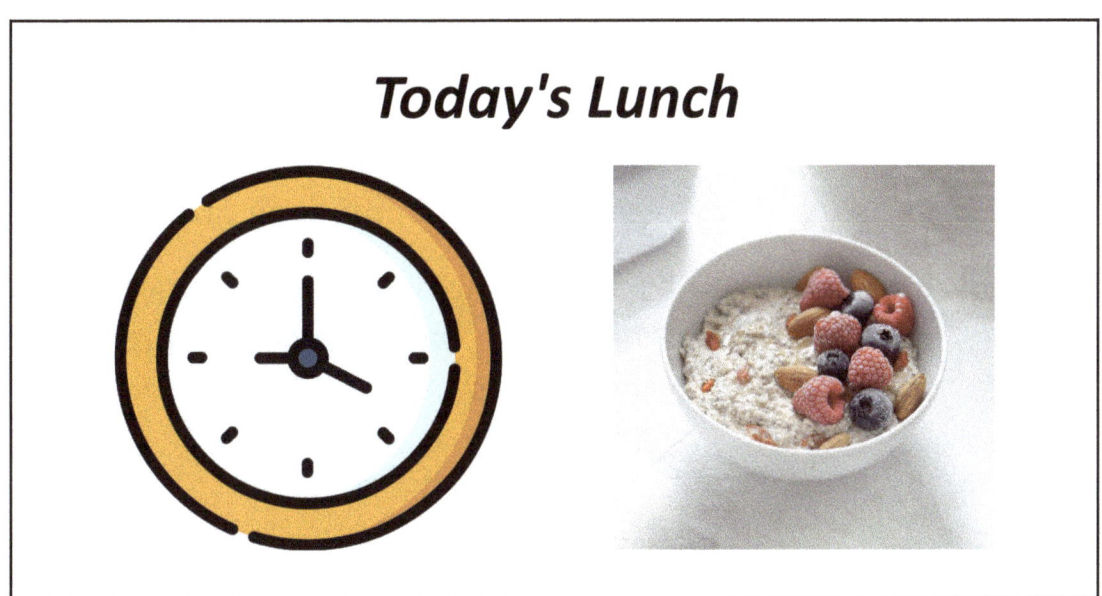

⋯→ *Implementation*

Stage 1: Modelling

Goal: Model appropriate self-feeding behavior for the child.

Token Economy

→ Used primarily to motivate child to learn to self-feed

→ Used to address issue of non-compliance of child with self-feeding

Modelling

→ Demonstrate to an inexperienced child the appropriate way of feeding oneself

→ Child learns new skill through modelling after an adult's actions

→ If child is unable to model successfully the adult's actions during initial attempts, use hand-over-hand prompts to guide the child's arm movements

⇢ *Implementation (continued)*

Stage 1: Modelling (continued)

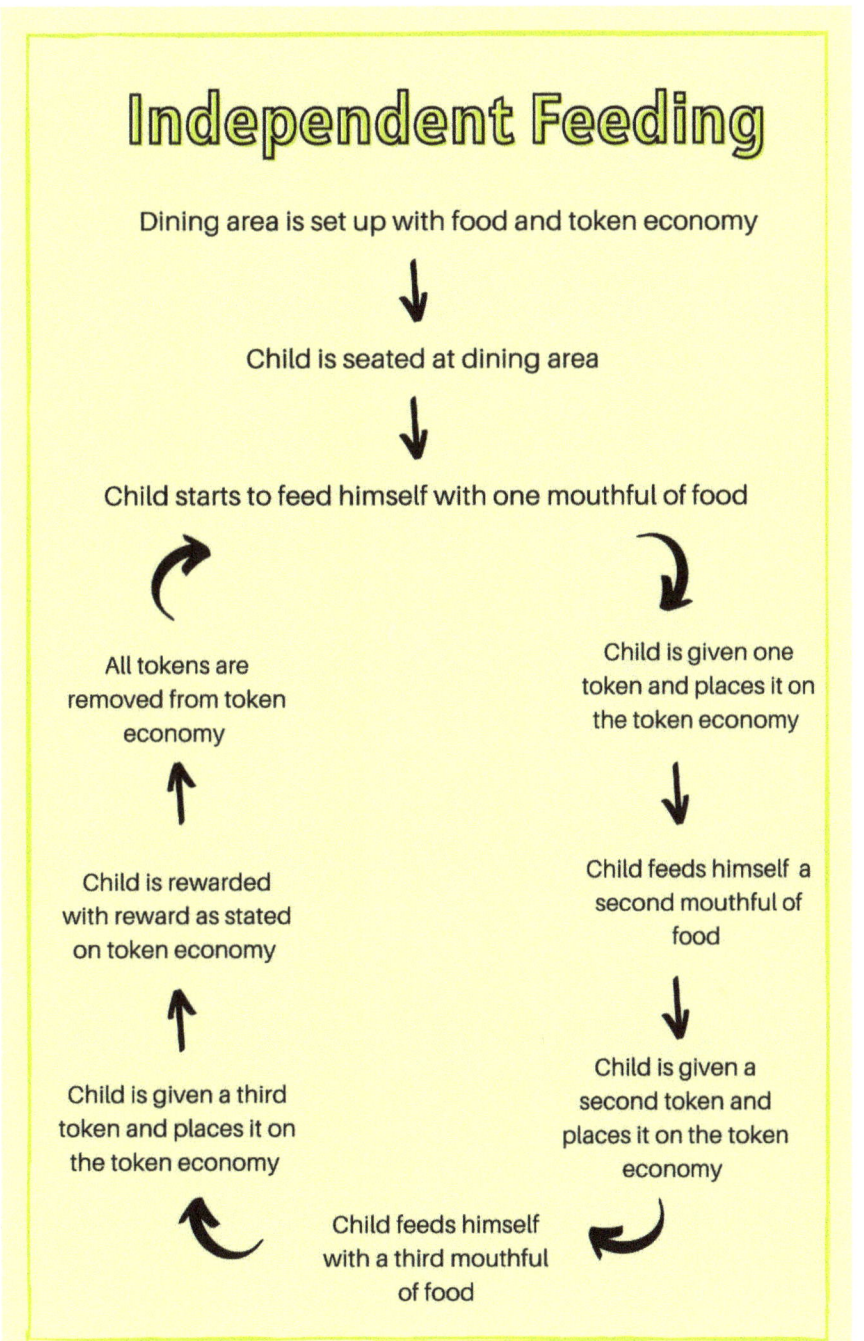

⸱⸱⸳→ *Implementation (continued)*

Stage 2: Independent feeding

Goal: Introduce child to different kinds of food and improve their nutritional intake

A number of children with autism tend to display restrictive and selective behaviors during eating (e.g., only eating certain kinds of food).

→ Increase frequency of reinforcement to increase the child's motivation

→ Increase the child's exposure to new type of food that will be introduced

→ Allow the child to lick, taste, smell, or touch the new type of food as much as the child wants

→ Never force a child to consume food that he or she is reluctant to try

⋯→ *Implementation (continued)*

Stage 2: Independent feeding (continued)

To introduce a different variety of food to the child, the type of food can be varied in terms of **color**, **texture**, and **solidity**. Start from what the child will eat in terms of texture and color, then scaffold to the targeted food.

Example:

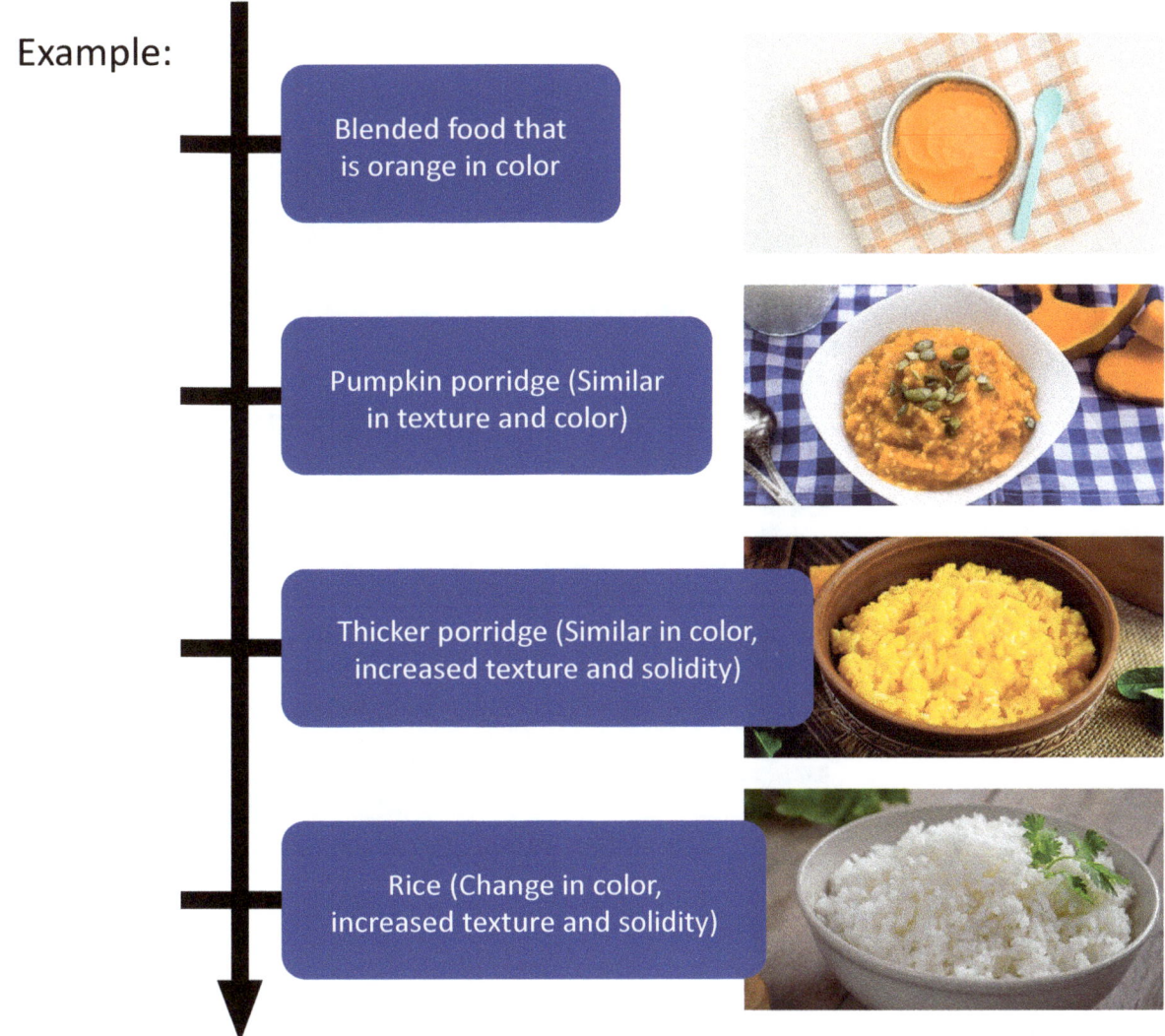

Blended food that is orange in color

Pumpkin porridge (Similar in texture and color)

Thicker porridge (Similar in color, increased texture and solidity)

Rice (Change in color, increased texture and solidity)

⋯→ *Implementation (continued)*

Stage 3: Fading away token economy system

Goal: Ensure that the child can independently self- feed without the need to be externally motivated by the token economy system

FADING PROCESS:

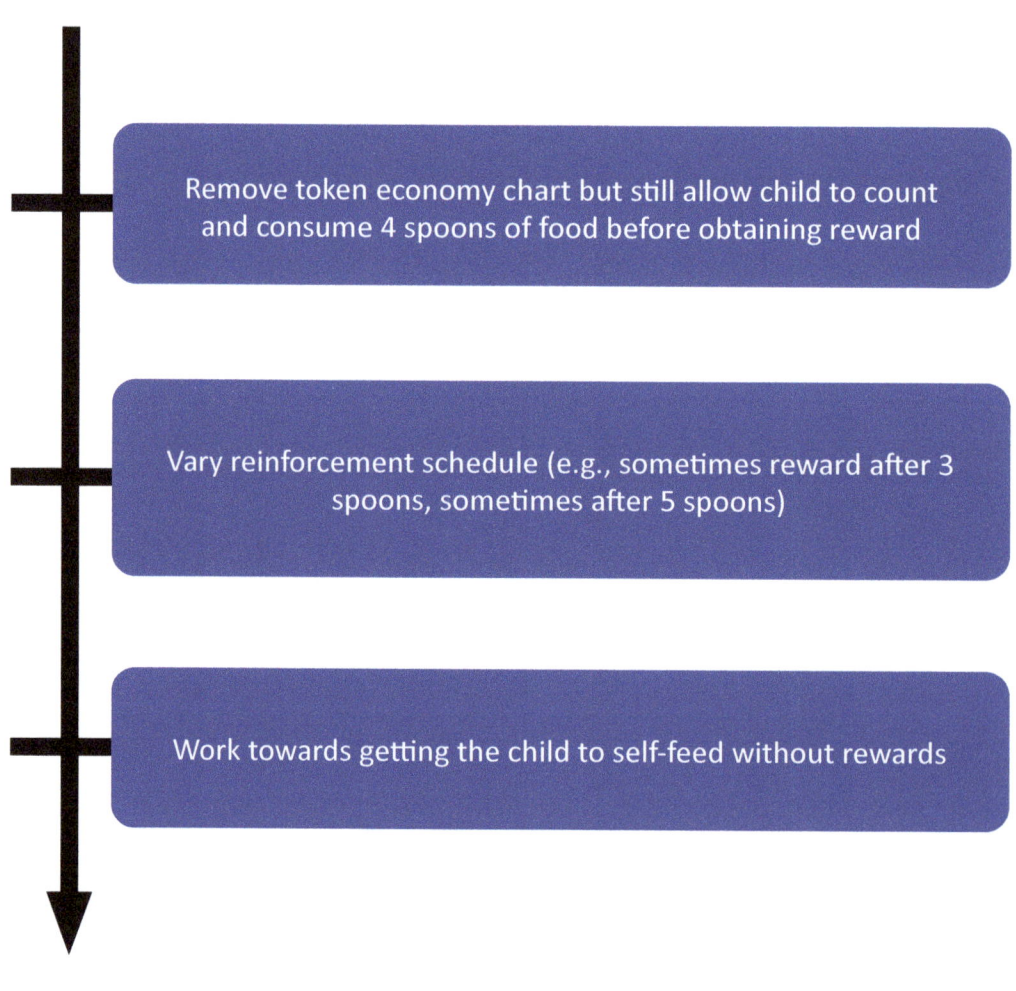

Remove token economy chart but still allow child to count and consume 4 spoons of food before obtaining reward

Vary reinforcement schedule (e.g., sometimes reward after 3 spoons, sometimes after 5 spoons)

Work towards getting the child to self-feed without rewards

⋯→ *Tips for feeding program*

✓ **Set behavioral expectations prior to feeding program**

E.g., through *Feeding Social Story*

TIME TO EAT!

My name is John.  *I need to eat every day.*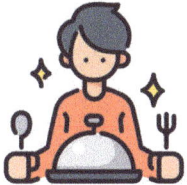

When I eat, I sit upright. 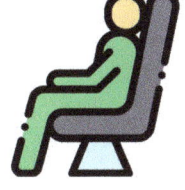 *I try my best to eat*

my food!  *Eating helps me become strong and*

healthy. 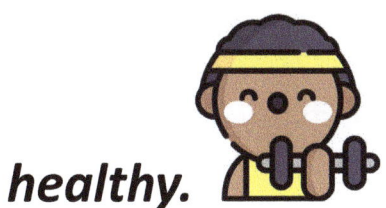 *I am a very good boy!*

┄→ *Tips for feeding program (continued)*

Set behavioral expectations prior to feeding program

✓ **Prepare softer and smaller food to facilitate consumption for children who have difficulty with chewing solid food**

> **E.g., cutting food into smaller pieces, cooking food longer to make it softer**

✓ **Supervise child to prevent accident**

> **Do NOT leave child alone, especially in the initial stages!**

✓ **Serve smaller portion of food during feeding program if child is unable to eat a normal portion when self-feeding**

> **The goal of the feeding program is to get child to eat a variety of food, and to train child to self-feed, NOT to get child to eat large amounts of food.**

✓ **Ensure that child is scooping an appropriate amount of food**

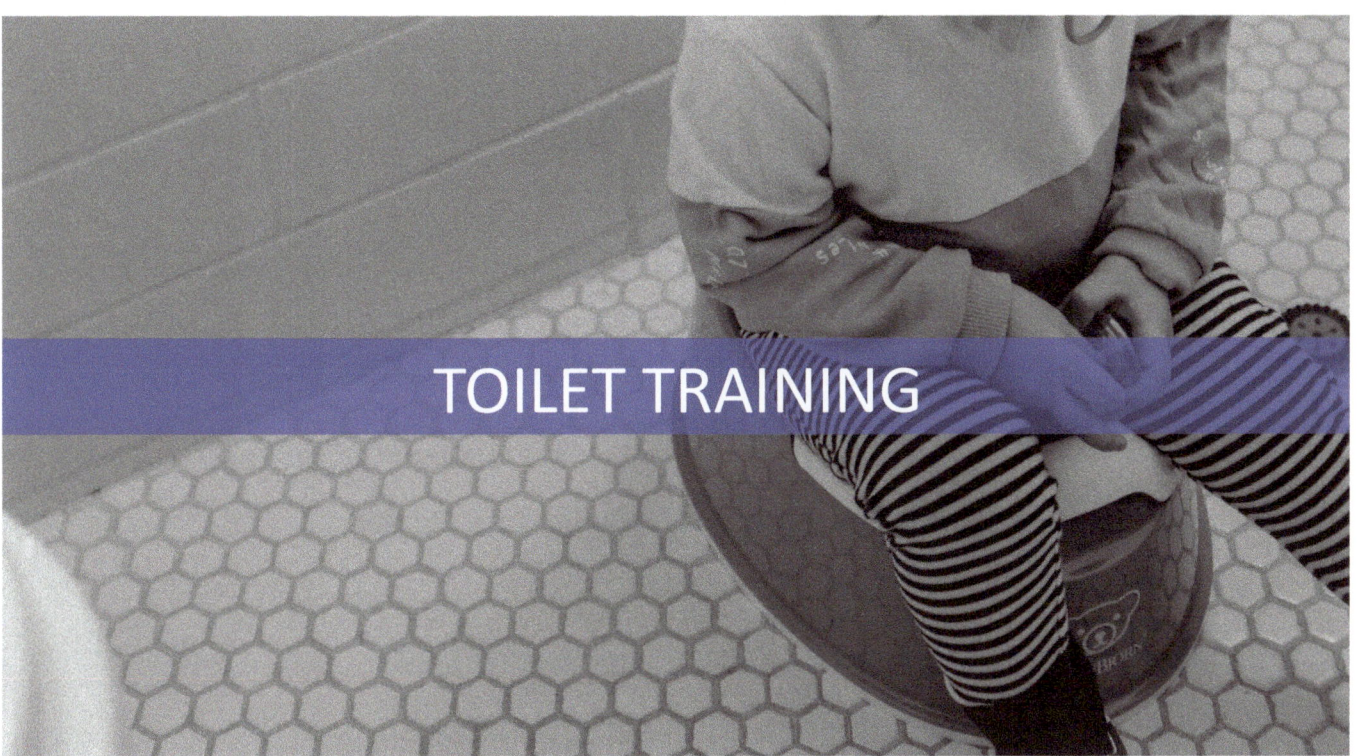

TOILET TRAINING

···→ *What is toilet training?*

- The training of a child to use the toilet for the purpose of urination and defecation

TOILET TRAINING

⋯→ *Assessing a child's readiness*

- Before starting to toilet-train the child, it is first necessary to determine if the child is ready for it.

- Parents can use the checklist below to assess the child's

- readiness:

Toilet Training Readiness Checklist

❑ Child has adequate finger and hand coordination

❑ Child is able to walk across room without assistance

❑ Child has bladder control—urinates a lot at once and does not dribble repeatedly (i.e., keeps diapers dry for 2 hours or more)

❑ Child is aware of the need to relieve oneself

❑ Child is able to understand and perform chaining of multiple steps

❑ Child is compliant and able to follow instructions

···→ *Preparation*

Gathering information

→ Map out child's schedule and determine preferred timings for toilet training

→ Note child's elimination habits (i.e., be aware of when the child usually urinates or defecates).

Preparing materials

Parents should prepare the following materials before beginning toilet-training

→ Loose-fitting shorts that are easy for the child to take off

→ Timer

→ Cloth or wet wipes for cleaning up

→ **Toilet routine (see page 92)**

→ **Toilet card (see page 93)**

→ **Reward chart (see page 94)**

→ Reward

⋯→ *Preparation (continued)*

Preparing materials (continued)

Toilet routine

➔ A toilet routine should be pasted on the toilet wall in a place where the child can refer to it easily.

Example:

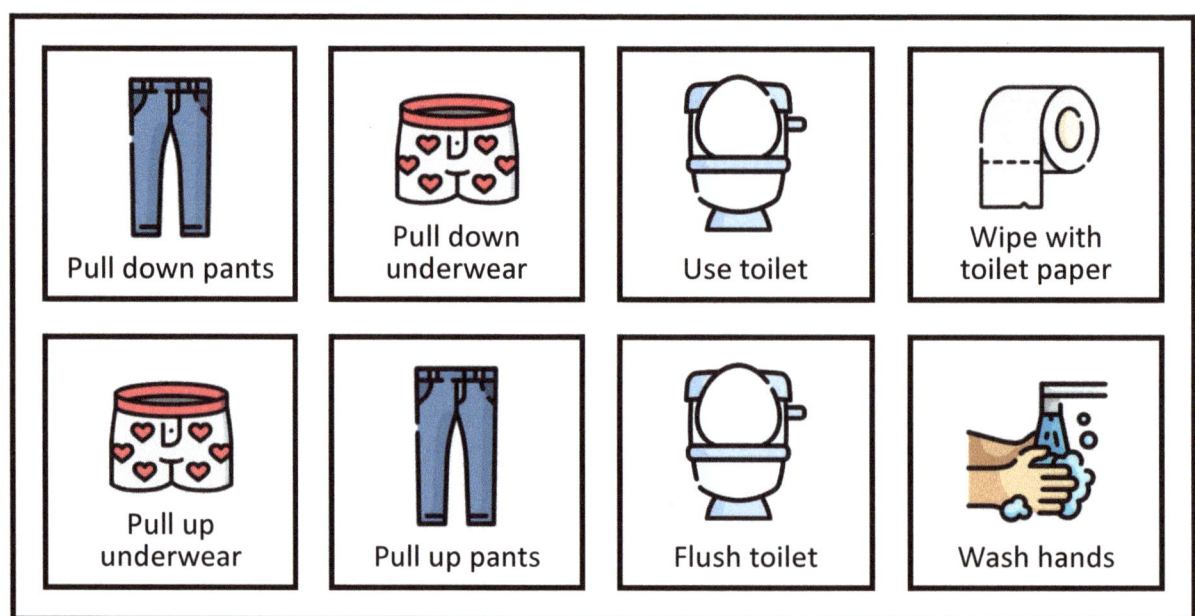

⋯→ *Preparation (continued)*

Preparing materials (continued)

Toilet requesting card

➔ A toilet requesting card is created for the child to express a need to go to the toilet.

Example:

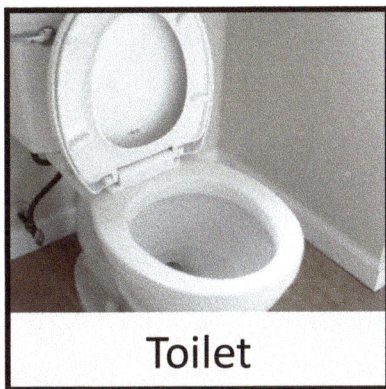

Toilet

➔ This card can either be pasted on the wall where the child can easily access it or hung onto the child's pants.

⋯→ *Preparation (continued)*

Preparing materials (continued)

Reward chart

➔ Parents should create a reward chart based on what the child likes.

➔ Reward chart should be pasted in front of the toilet bowl or in a place the child can see when sitting on the potty/toilet bowl.

Example:

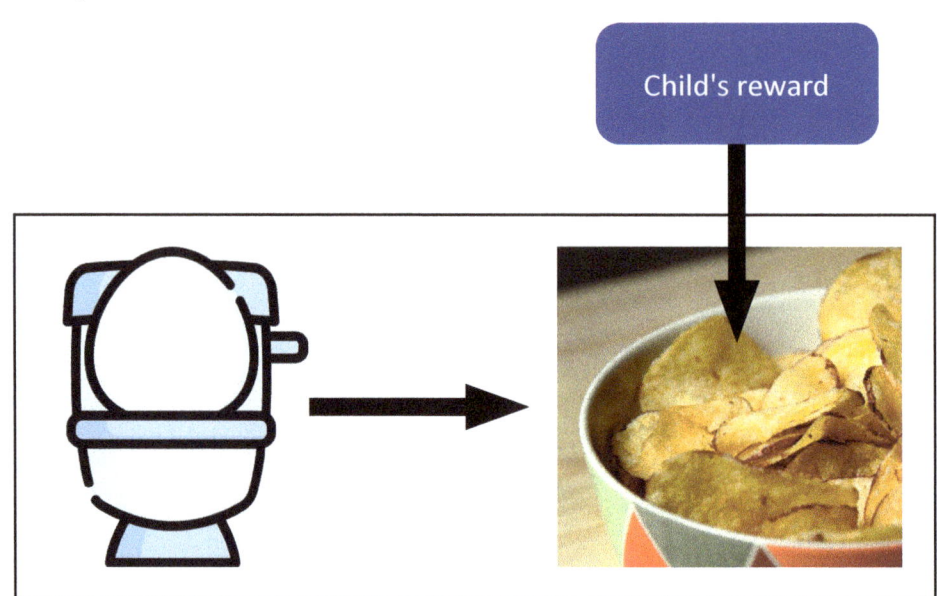

···→ *Implementation*

Hydration

→ It is important to get the child to drink a lot of water during the toilet-training process.

→ This is because when the child drinks more water, it creates opportunities to urinate, which in turn creates opportunities to reinforce appropriate elimination.

Scheduled sittings

→ Child is brought to the bathroom at regular intervals.

→ Intervals are predetermined and will usually be around every 30 minutes at the start.

→ Intervals may be shortened in periods when the child will likely eliminate.

→ Parents can set a timer (e.g., 30 minutes) to indicate that it is time to go to the toilet.

⋯→ *Implementation (continued)*

Scheduled Sitting (continued)

Once the timer rings, parent and child go through the following:

1. Child picks up the "toilet card" and gives it to the parents (requesting)

2. Parent brings child to the toilet

3. Child follows the steps on the toilet routine

4. Parent gets child to sit on toilet bowl for 5 minutes

5. If child eliminates, parent gives praise and reward instantly, and child continues with rest of toilet routine

6. If child does not eliminate, child completes the rest of the toilet routine after time is up

7. Child continues daily activities. Parent sets timer again to schedule another toilet break.

⟶ *Implementation (continued)*

③ Weaning

→ After child manages successful toileting with no accidents for several days, parents can start weaning off the training.

→ Instead of setting a timer, parents wait for child to request or to go to the toilet by himself.

④ Generalization

→ After successfully toilet-training at home, parents can generalize that skill to other toilets (e.g., school toilets, toilet at shopping malls)

→ It's good to have a toilet routine handy (e.g., on phone) if the child still needs the routine.

⋯→ *Accident procedure*

(What to do if the child eliminates outside of the bathroom)

If a child eliminates outside of the bathroom, parents are to follow the following steps:

1. Give verbal disapproval (a flat "no)

2. Parents prompt from the back to get child to initiate cleaning up process

   → Child changes into new set of clothes

   → Child cleans up the mess created

   → Child HAS to be involved in the cleaning process (natural corrective action)

3. Continue daily activities after cleaning

⋯→ *Accident procedure (continued)*

(What to do if the child eliminates outside of the bathroom)

- Use hand-over-hand from behind the child to perform the cleaning if necessary.

- Do not scold the child or show signs of exasperation.

- Do not nag at the child and try to maintain silence during the whole procedure.

- Prepare materials needed for accident management beforehand to facilitate the procedure (i.e., keep a spare set of clothes and clean-up rag near the child's activity station).

- Do not make the cleaning enjoyable for the child; any stereotypical or maladaptive behaviors should be restricted or blocked.

⋯→ *Tips for toilet-training*

✓ Many children with autism have accompanying sensory disorders resulting in unusual reactions to smells, sights, or sounds associated with the bathroom or its use.

✓ Do not punish or scold the child should accidents happen or when the child does not want to sit for the required period of time.

✓ Identify powerful reinforcers and keep them as such (withholding them from the child for a period of time prior to the training) so that they can be effectively used for successful elimination by the child.

✓ Stick by the schedule that was predetermined and follow through with it.

✓ Do not allow the child to wear diapers once training commences except during nighttime or naptime.

Chapter 5

SMALL GROUP INTERVENTION

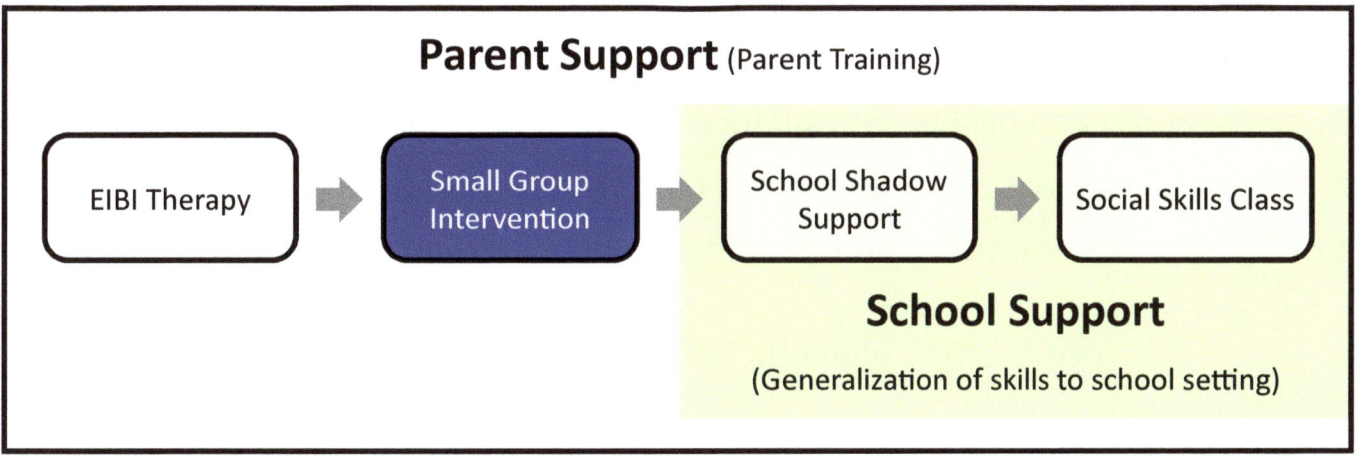

The next stage of the CMEI model is Small Group Intervention.

At this stage, the child starts joining other children of similar abilities to learn and develop in a safe setting under the guidance of therapists.

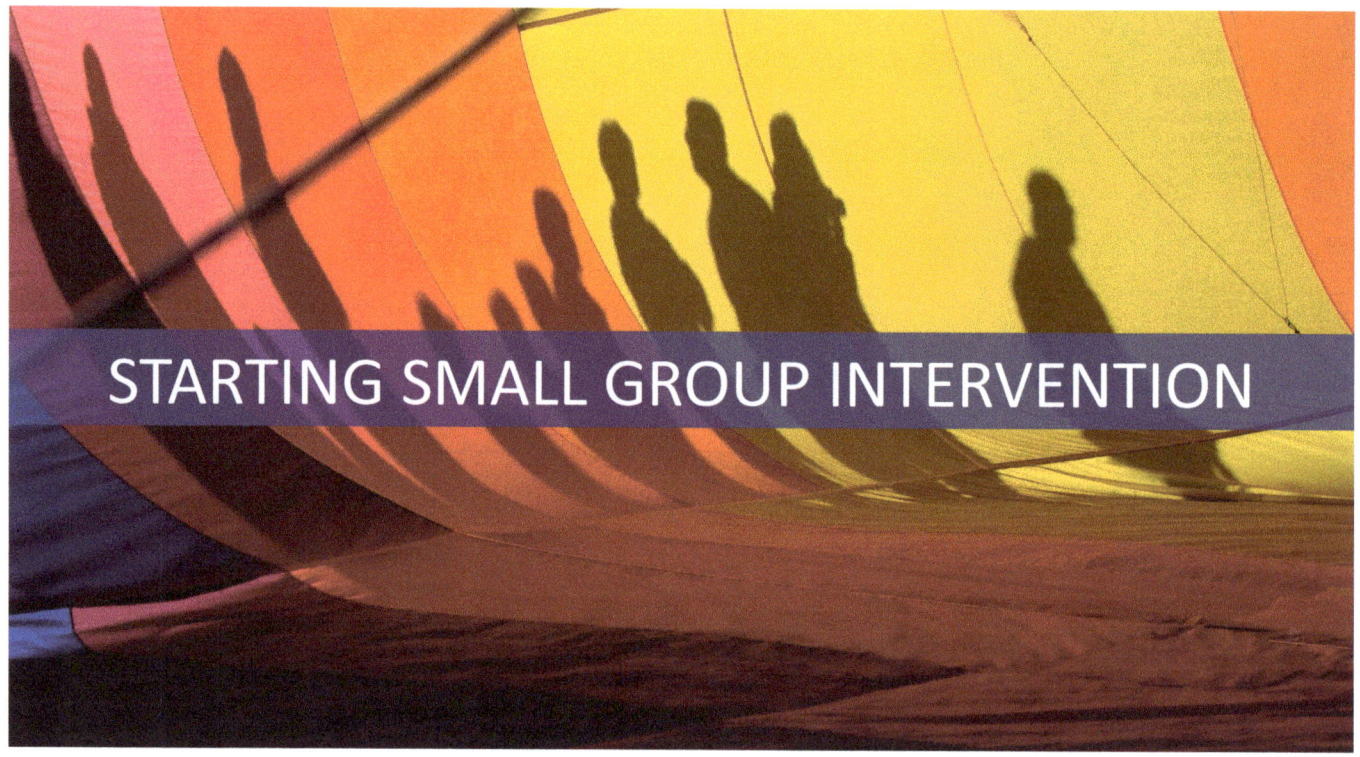

STARTING SMALL GROUP INTERVENTION

Once the child establishes compliance in a one-to-one setting, it is important for the child to start generalizing this compliance to a small group setting. For small group intervention, the following approaches can be used:

1. Structured Teaching by Division (TEACCH)

2. Activity-based approach to intervention or routine-based intervention

3. Behavioral reinforcement using token economy and group contingency

STRUCTURED TEACHING

···→ *What is structured teaching?*

Structured teaching is a therapeutic tool which was devised by Division TE-ACCH at the University of North Carolina at Chapel Hill to help individuals with ASD understand their surroundings and improve their learning based on the information that they take in. The approach emphasizes the structure and organization of the learning environment—physical setup, learning materials, and instructional foci.

This approach relies on five basic principles, which are represented in the form of a pyramid. The principle at the bottom is the most important one; it lays the foundation in the design of the structured teaching classroom.

Visual Structure of Materials

Routines and Visual Strategies

Work Systems

Schedules

A pyramid hierarchy model of structured teaching principles

Physical Structure

⋯→ *Physical Structure*

Physical structure is used in the classroom environment to help the children understand the expectations of the respective area. It also provides meaning to the environment, as each area is specifically set up to encourage desirable habits. When the children are able to understand the expectations of each learning area, they will be able to manage their sensory stimulation and regulate their behaviors better. Good self-regulation helps children focus better on tasks until completion. A structured teaching classroom can be clearly set up using boards and colored tapes and/or by making out areas.

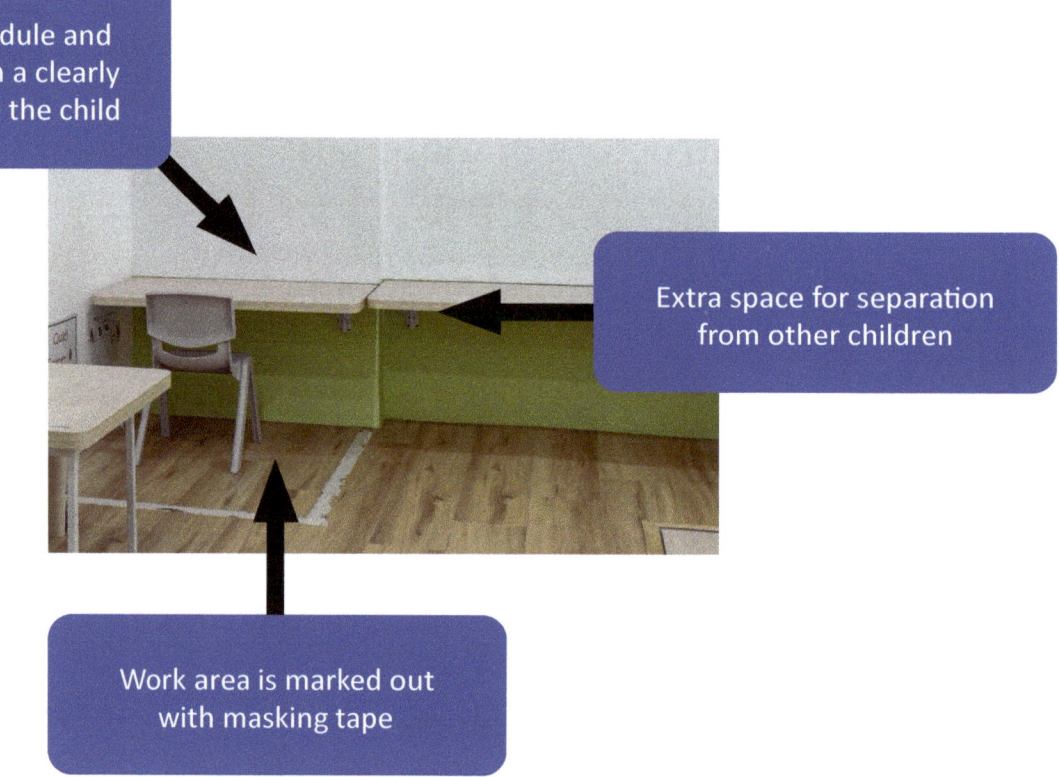

Can put task schedule and token economy on a clearly visible spot before the child

Extra space for separation from other children

Work area is marked out with masking tape

⋯→ *Physical Structure (continued)*

In order to create a structured environment, specific areas for different activities should be marked:

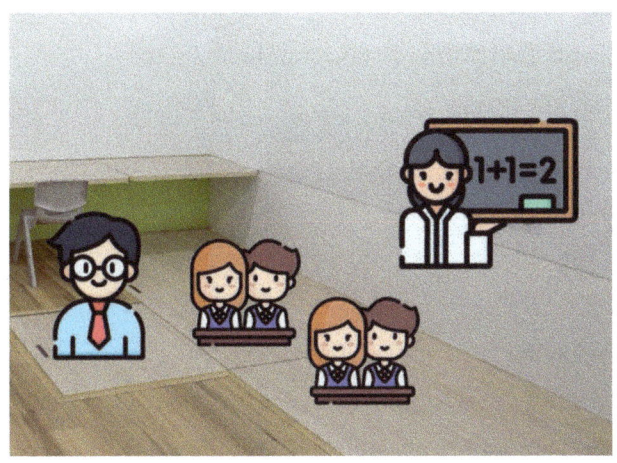

Small group activity

Lessons typically begin with a small group activity (e.g., circle time, story reading), and at times, related activities are conducted (e.g., art, music) in which children are expected to learn to share space and materials. In groups of five children maximum, the children are seated side by side in a semi-circle arrangement with the lead therapist facing all children. The support therapist will be seated behind the children to provide the relevant prompts to the children to remind them to stay seated while the session is ongoing. This will minimize disruption to the therapist who is anchoring the session.

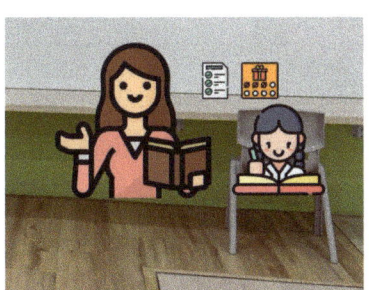

Work with therapist (one-to-one)

This set-up is particularly useful in teaching skills which require a lot of guidance (e.g., work habits, problem-solving, motor-planning) or tasks which the children are newly exposed to. The child will sit facing the board to minimize disruption, and the teacher will usually sit to the left of the child. Tasks are presented from left to right.

⋯→ *Physical Structure (continued)*

In order to create a structured environment, specific areas for different activities should be marked:

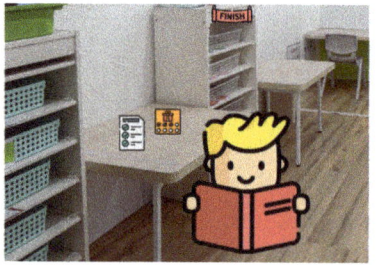 **Independent work area**	In this area, familiar tasks are arranged in order (left to right; top to down) on a shelf to the left of the table. The child is required to complete each task in sequence. There is no direct teaching involved apart from prompting the child to: • Take tasks • Complete tasks • Keep task by placing it either on the shelf or in the finished basket
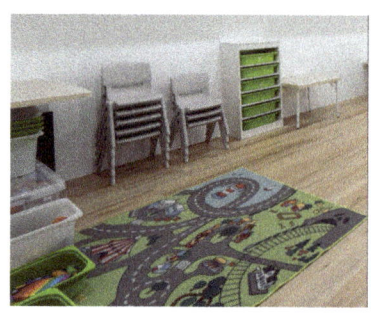 **Play area**	This area is set up for children to develop their play skills, which is usually done through facilitation from the therapist. The toys are placed in trays based on their theme or function. Children are encouraged to sit on the mat so they can explore various types of toys and setups. Children may be exposed to the following types of play: • Structured play • Guided play • Free play
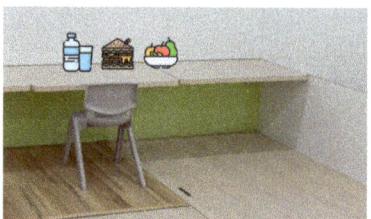 **Snack area**	This area is clearly located with visuals, and children are required to bring their water bottles and snack box to their respective seating areas around the table. During snack time, children are required to practice their communication skills, such as requesting using either verbal skills or their augmentative communication tools (e.g.,PECS).

⋯→ *Visual schedules*

A visual schedule serves as a timetable for children. It depicts a specific activity, its location, and the person the child will be working with. Basically, it tells the child WHEN to do the activity, as the visual sequence of the activities are arranged in a top-down manner on a board. A transition object (e.g., image of the child or interest object) is used to help the child understand that it is time to check the schedule. There are three types of schedules:

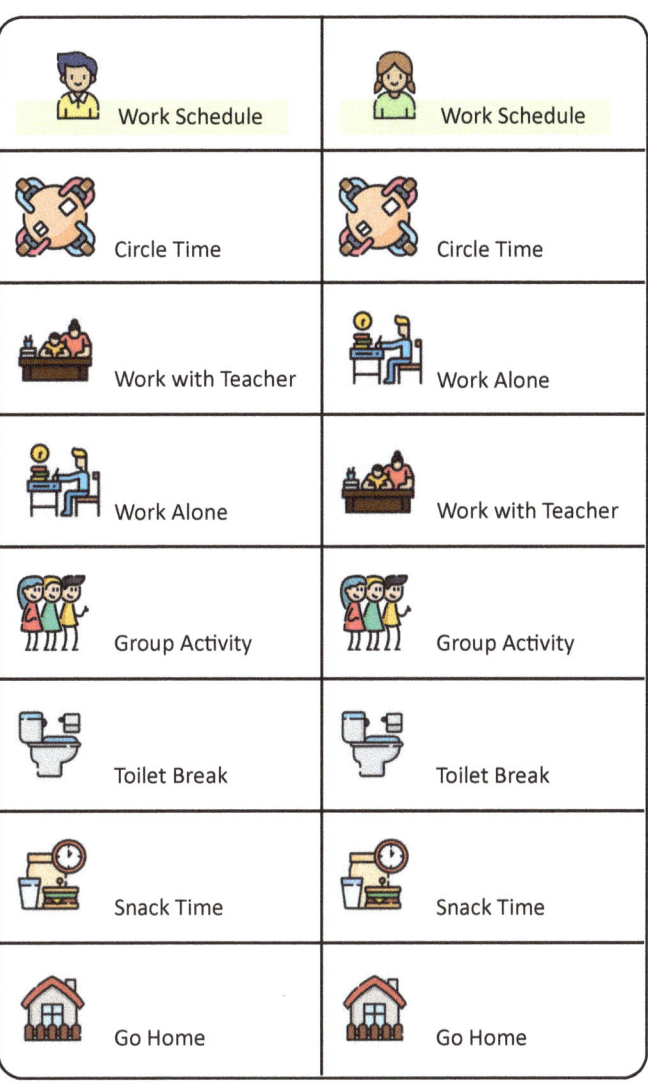

- *First-then:* Two pictures to teach the child the simple sequence of activities.

- *Half-session:* Usually four to five activities depicted to represent an hour-and-a-half time frame.

- *Full-session:* Up to eight to ten activities are depicted to represent a three-hour time frame.

 ## *Visual schedules (continued)*

Levels of visual presentation

Concrete

Objects Things associated with the venue or activity (e.g., toilet roll = toilet; favorite piece of puzzle = work with teacher; snack box = snack time)	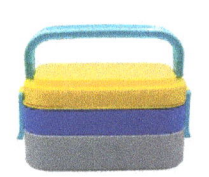
Photos Examples include photos of self or of favorite item, location, or activity. Words may be used to associate the relevant meanings with items.	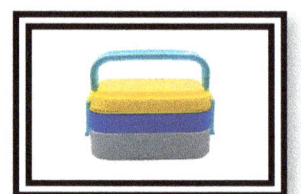
Pictures/drawings Depictions of interest or easily recalled items which clearly represent the associated activity. Words are usually introduced too.	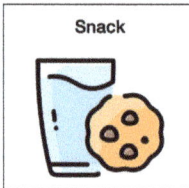
Written words Associated words are typed or written. The child checks the associated word after reading by checking them off or removing them from the schedule.	**snack**

Abstract

┅➤ *Visual schedules (continued)*

How can I implement a schedule?

 **Pre-implementation**

- Determine the transition material that the child needs (e.g., object, photos, pictures, words)

- Determine the type or level of visual presentation that the child needs

- Determine the length of the schedule; the child will be using a first-then, half-session, or full-session schedule

- Determine the size of visual presentation (image & font) that the child responds to

⋯→ *Visual schedules (continued)*

How can I implement a schedule?

 **2** **During implementation**

→ Pass the "transition object" (e.g., 'check schedule' card) to the child

→ Paste the "transition object" on the respective schedule and take out the activity card (prompt from behind, use gestural or physical prompt, fade the prompt subsequently)

→ Find the locator and paste the activity card on it

→ Upon completion, repeat above steps

If the child can proceed to the check schedule area **voluntarily** upon completion of each activity, it is okay to not pass him the "check schedule" card

Example of "check schedule" card

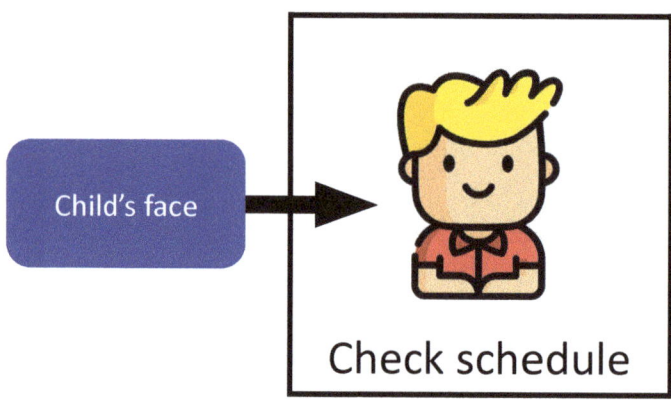

Child's face → Check schedule

⋯→ *Visual schedules (continued)*

How can I implement a schedule?

Post-implementation

Check for the following behaviors from the child:

→ Looks at the activity card and looks for the locator

→ Knows what to do after putting the visual card on the locator—doing what the card says (e.g., sit down on chair for circle time)

→ **Does not** move to the location before checking the visual schedule (meaning the child has memorized the routine and changes need to be introduced)

→ Displays readiness to move on to the next level of visual representation (more abstract)

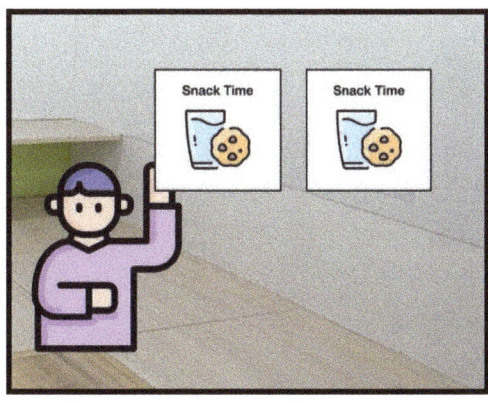

Child matches activity card with locator

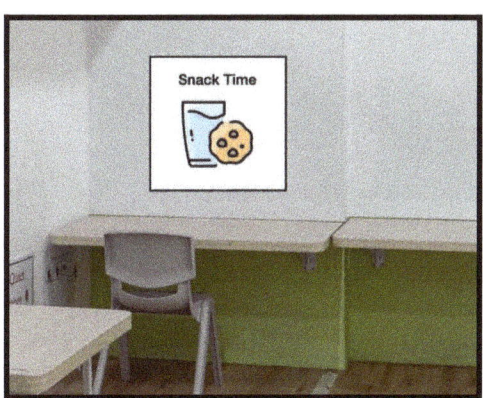

Locator placed directly where the child is supposed to be

┈→ *Work system*

What is a work system?

A work system serves as a to-do-list for children. It tells the child

- **What** should I do?

- **How much** work needs to be done?

- **How do** I know when I'm finished?

- **What** do I do next?

When is a work system used with children?

A work system is used during the following sessions:

- Independent task: Child has to complete an array of 4- 6 tasks independently

- Work with therapist: Child works with therapist on 1-1 basis

⋯→ *Work system (continued)*

How can I implement a schedule?

Pre-implementation

Determine the number of tasks to be completed during the duration of the session (20-30min)

- For a child who is new to the system, start off with 2 tasks (first-then system)

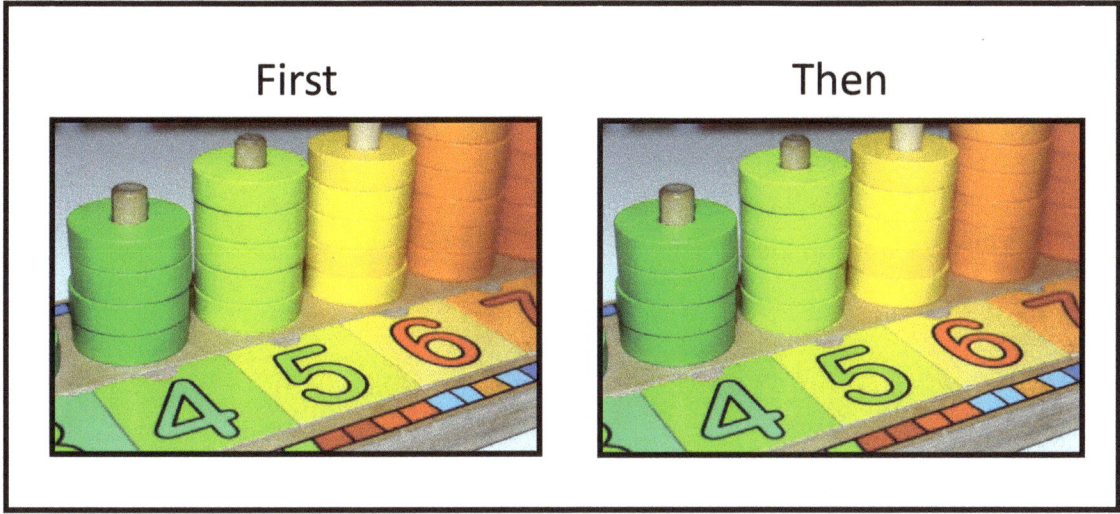

- For a child who is more familiar, between 4-5 tasks can be introduced apart from the motivational task

- Tasks should contain a combination of the domains—cognitive, fine-motor, language, adaptive skills

⋯→ *Work system (continued)*

Pre-implementation (continued)

An example of a setup for independent work:

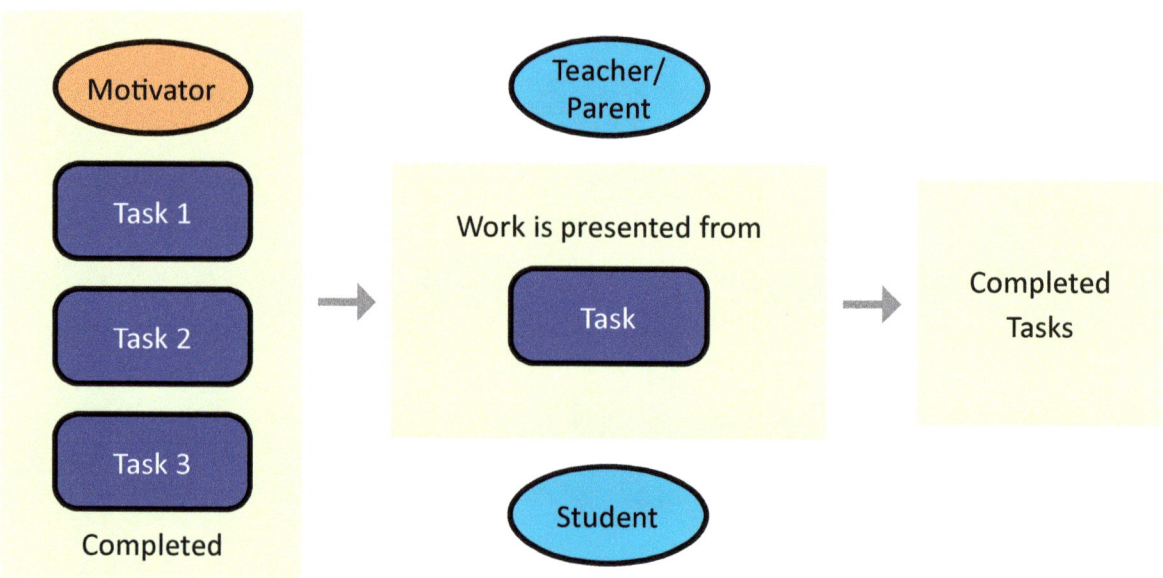

⋯→ *Work system (continued)*

During implementation

- Pass the "transition object" (e.g., "check schedule" card) to the child. Move the child to the "work with teacher" station

- Paste the "work with teacher" card on the locator

- Greet the child and make sure the child is ready for work

- Show the work system for the tasks and read through once (point accordingly) to the child

- Present the task to the child (if the child can take the task on his own, get the child to do it independently). Prompt the child when necessary

- Demonstrate the start of the task and get the child to complete independently

- Praise the child enthusiastically when the child gets it correct and completes the task

- Direct the child to put the task away into the finish basket

- Repeat until all tasks are completed

···▸ *Work system (continued)*

3 **Post-implementation**

Check for the following from the child:

- Matches the visuals on the work system to the correct task

- Knows that he/she needs to start working on the task after removing it from the shelf

- Performs the correct sequence of tasks

	 Work Schedule	✓
1	Circle Time	◯
2	Work Alone	◯
3	Work with Teacher	◯
4	Group Activity	◯
5	Toilet Break	◯
6	Snack Time	◯
7	Go Home	◯

A visual work system which uses a "tick" to check the completed task

⋯→ *Routine*

Routines are useful to ensure predictability and minimizes anxiety for the children during the session. Routines are created for tasks that the child is required to do in a fixed order **all the time**.

Steps for using a routine:

① Create a visual-based routine and paste it on

➔ Routine should be pasted where the child is expected to complete the routine (E.g., toilet routine pasted near the toilet)

② Learning of routine

➔ Initially, therapist should use hand-over-hand to guide the child step by step, pointing to the steps on the routine

③ Fading of routine

➔ Once child is familiarized, child refers to routine by himself without adult prompt

⋯→ *Routine (continued)*

Example:

ARRIVAL ROUTINE

1	Shoes in cubby hole	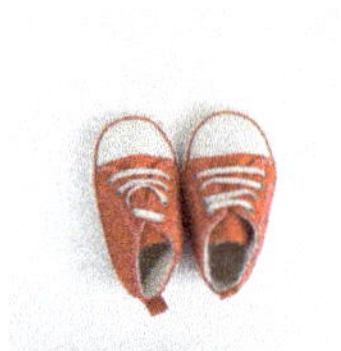
2	Snack in cubby hole	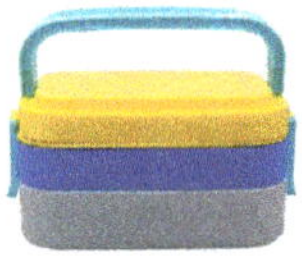
3	Bag in cubby hole	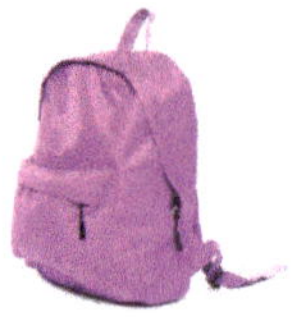
4	Take temperature	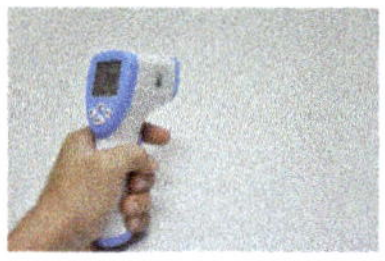
5	Sanitize hands	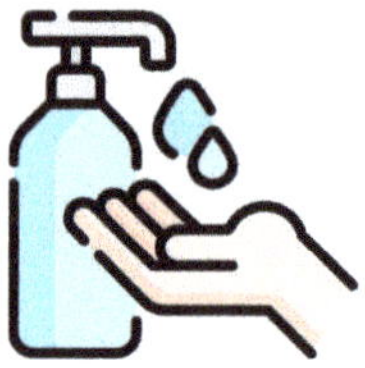

···→ *What is positive behavior reinforcement?*

Reinforcement is the process in which a behavior is strengthened by the immediate consequence that reliably follows its occurrence. To "strengthen" a behavior is to make it occur more frequently, meaning the child is exposed more to the desired consequence following an appropriate behavior. Positive behavior reinforcement is part of Applied Behavior Analysis, in which a child's behavior is conditioned by a desired reinforcer. There are two types of reinforcers: primary and secondary. A primary reinforcer is a concrete item (e.g., toy, food) or favorite activity which the child is immediately exposed to following an appropriate behavior. A secondary reinforcer is a conditioned set of items (e.g., tokens) which the child needs to accumulate to exchange for the primary reinforcer.

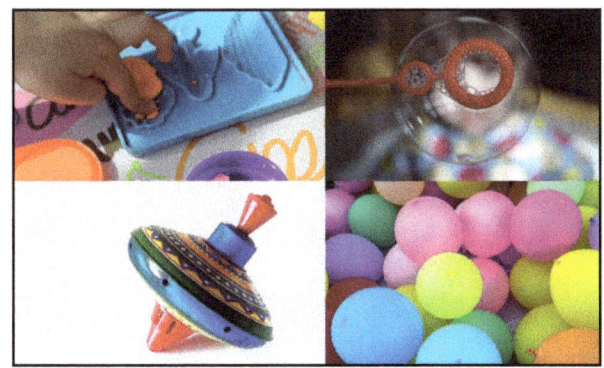

Choices of primary reinforcers may include spinning tops, balloons, bubbles to gain attention and motivation of children

⋯→ *Token Economy*

The token economy used during small group intervention is the same as the token economy used for EIBI (stage 1 of CMEI). More information on how to use it can be found on page 16.

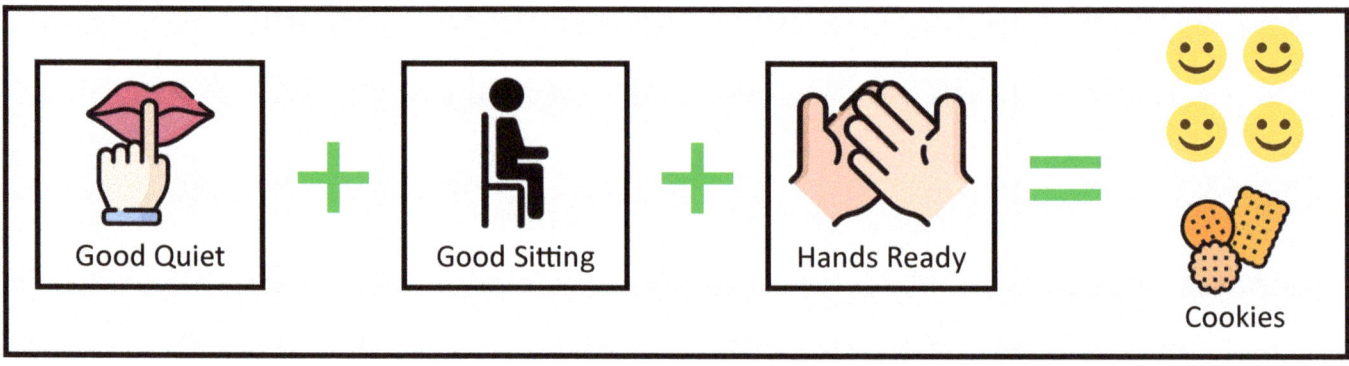

Goals can be changed to suit behavioral needs in small group intervention.

···→ *Group-oriented contingency system*

A group-oriented contingency is when an entire class is reinforced based on the behavior of one student, a number of students, or the entire class. Children with higher ability will be exposed to the group contingency system in which they will accumulate tokens for the class which can be exchanged for a common favorite activity, a song, or even a video clip. Each student earns the reward (token) based on their own behavior, and no student is penalized for the behavior of anyone else. This will encourage children to learn appropriate behavior from peers quickly.

How do we prepare a group contingency system?

The trick to effective positive reinforcement is finding what is truly reinforcing to children. Therapists are encouraged to prepare a basket of different reinforcers for children to select from, as the reinforcer may lose its strength over time. Therapists can determine what is positively reinforcing to the children by simply watching what activities children choose when they have free access to do whatever they want or what they do often.

⋯→ *Group-oriented contingency system (continued)*

Example of a group contingency system chart:

TOKEN EXCHANGE SYSTEM

1 token	4 tokens	8 tokens	10 tokens

···→ *Prompting hierarchy*

Prompting hierarchies provide a systematic method of assisting students to learn and use new skills, as well as a framework for therapists to communicate about a child's learning and level of independence. The method is also called the levels of prompt, meaning children are provided with various levels of prompt ranging from the most intrusive (full physical prompt) to the least intrusive (natural cue).

Full physical assistance

Partial physical

Modeling

Gesture

Verbal

Independent

⋯→ *Prompting hierarchy*

Guidelines for administering prompts:

- Always remember that prompts are to help the child cope better.

- Allow 3-5 seconds between each prompt to allow the child to process and respond appropriately.

- Always start from less intrusive prompts—ONLY move up when the child still can't achieve it.

- Move to less intrusive prompts when the child achieves basic levels of a task.

- Therapist can pair up different prompts and slowly fade off the prompts. (E.g., Verbal + gesture ➜ Gestural ➜ Visual)

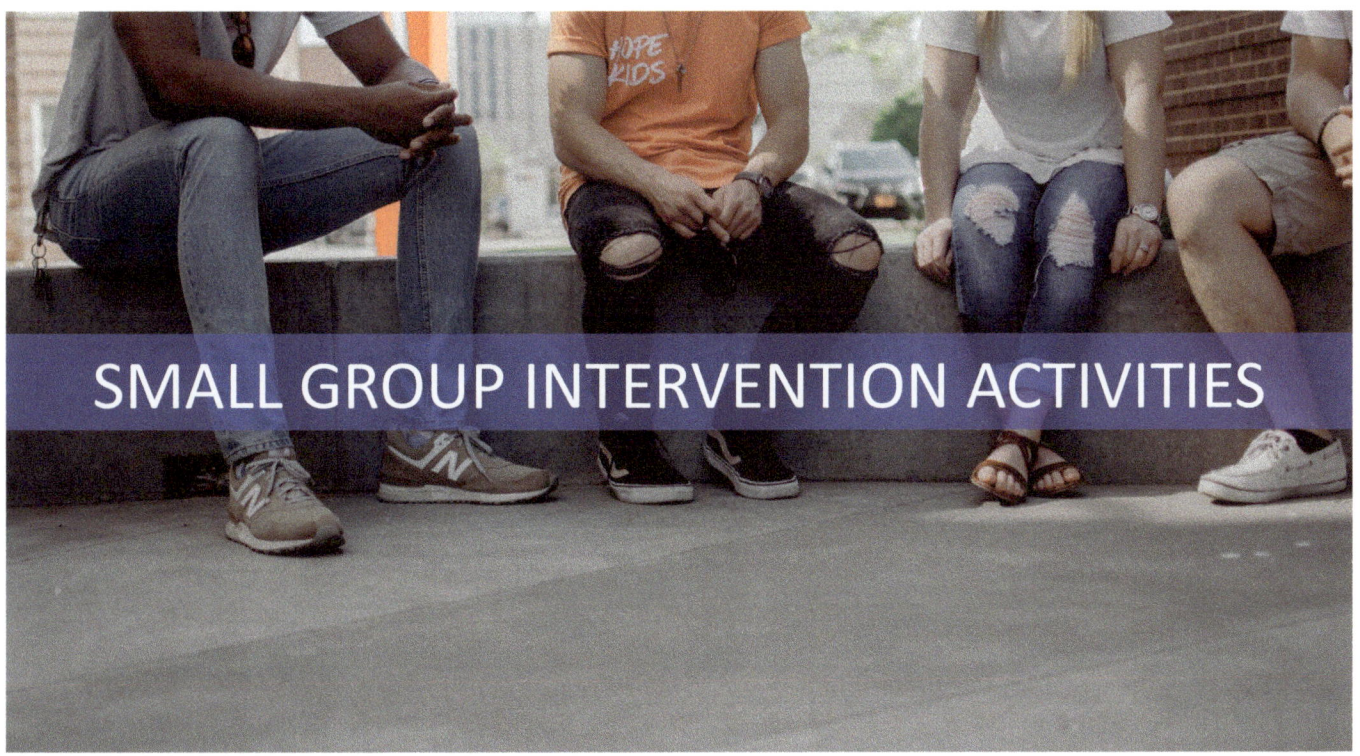

SMALL GROUP INTERVENTION ACTIVITIES

In this section, a typical small group intervention session will be described in detail. Therapists should change or adapt activities based on the child. Smooth transition between activities is crucial, as many children with autism tend to face challenges with transition. Therefore, between activities, it is important for therapists to get the child to check the schedule using the "check schedule" card or by finding locators.

Arrival of child

Once child arrives, child completes the arrival routine (guided by therapist initially).

ARRIVAL ROUTINE

1	**Shoes in cubby hole**	
2	**Snack in cubby hole**	
3	**Bag in cubby hole**	
4	**Take temperature**	
5	**Sanitize hands**	

Circle Time

The first activity for the therapy session can be circle time, in which greetings, attendance-taking, and social interaction take place.

A typical circle time covers the following aspects:

➜ Greetings to teachers and peers

➜ Checking of attendance

➜ Making choices of activities (e.g., songs, stories) using choice board

➜ Understanding spatial concept (time, date)

➜ Making predictions (e.g., weather forecast)

➜ Show and tell

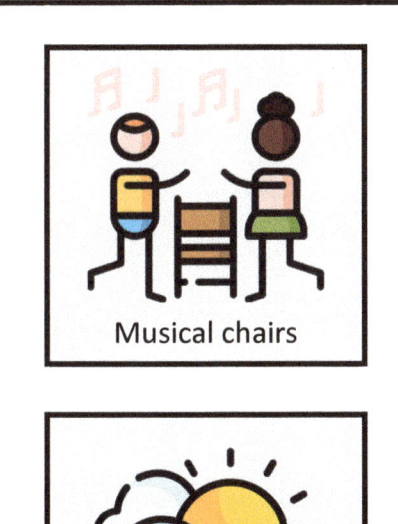

Musical chairs

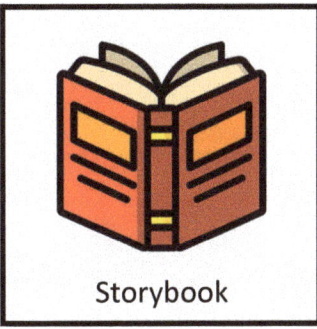

Storybook

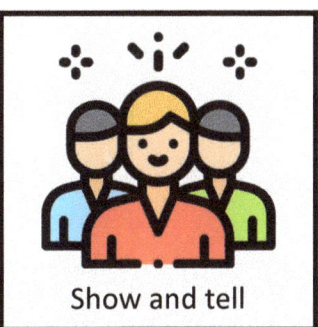

Show and tell

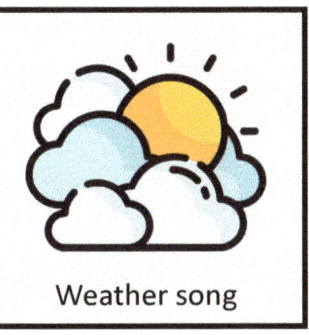

Weather song

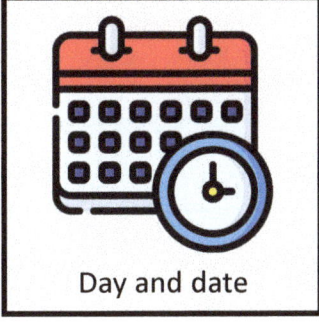

Day and date

Example of choice board—children take turns to choose an activity

3 Work with teacher/individual work

Transition: After circle time, therapist passes child the "check schedule" card to transition child to the next activity.

- During work with teacher/individual work time, child completes tasks according to a schedule (one-on-one with a therapist or independently)

- Tasks involved include numeracy, literacy, motor skill, and visuospatial tasks (further details in Chapter 3: EIBI)

- Child follows the schedule and checks off tasks accordingly.

	Work Schedule	✓
1	Circle Time	◯
2	Work Alone	◯
3	Work with Teacher	◯
4	Group Activity	◯
5	Toilet Break	◯
6	Snack Time	◯
7	Go Home	◯

Example of task schedule

Toilet break

Toilet breaks are scheduled at frequent intervals to help children get accustomed to the routine. During toilet breaks as a class, children will do the following:

Use "check schedule" card to identify the activity card "toilet"

Line up in a row

Wait for turn to go toilet

During child's turn, paste the toilet card on the locator and go in the toilet

Follow toilet routine (Page 92)

Return to class and wait for friends

Structured play

As many children with autism do not naturally learn to play and communicate with their peers, structured play is also conducted during small group interventions, with the aim of allowing the children to play together under the guidance of therapists. During play, the therapist guides the child to interact with other children (e.g., asking peers to share toys with them, take turns, or initiate playing together with peers). Example of structured play activities include sand play, water play, and playing with blocks.

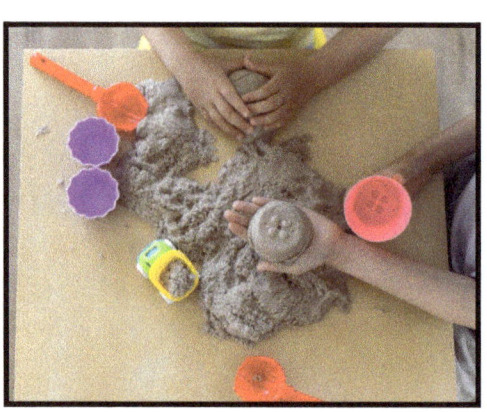

Indoor sand play

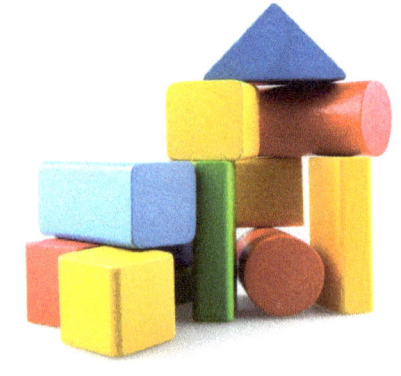

Playing with blocks

Snack time

The goal of snack time is to train the child for independent self-feeding, training the child for mainstream preschools or primary schools.

During snack time, the child goes through the following steps:

Child pastes "snack time" card on the locator

Take snack from tray and proceed to seat

Keep snack box into bag after eating

Wash hands

Return to class and get ready for next activity

Departure of child

Child follows a departure routine:

DEPARTURE ROUTINE

1	Sing "goodbye" song	
2	Take bag	
3	Wear shoes	
4	Say "bye" to teacher	

Chapter 6

SCHOOL SHADOW SUPPORT

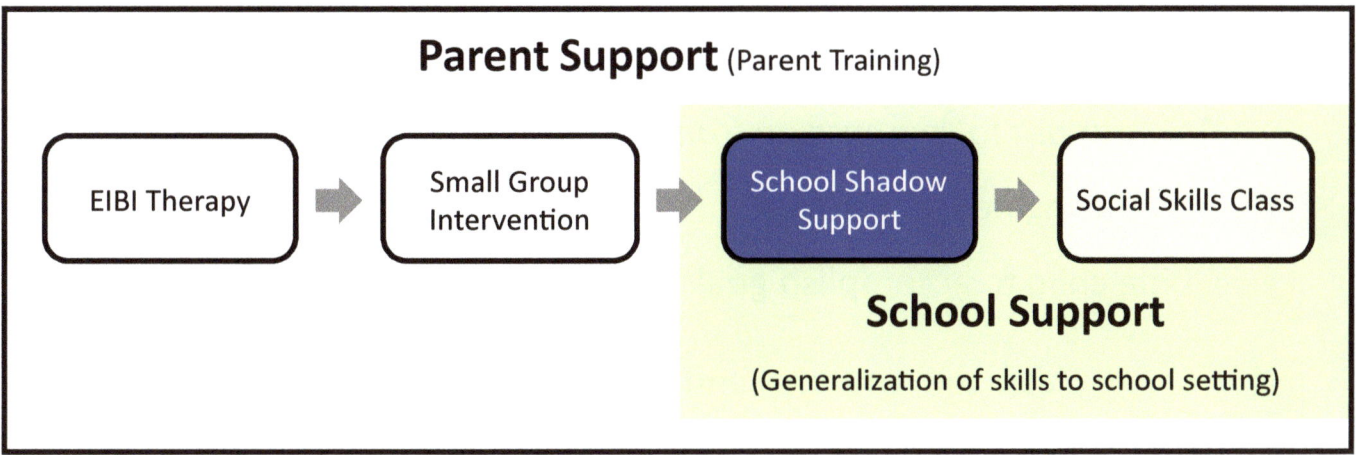

The next stage of the CMEI model is School Shadow Support.

At this stage, child joins a mainstream preschool or primary school (depending on age), accompanied by a shadow teacher.

⋯→ *What is school shadow support?*

School shadow support is the provision of one-to-one guidance for a child in a mainstream school setting. The child attends lessons like the other children in the class, guided by a shadow teacher.

⋯→ *Role of the shadow teacher*

- Key role: help child assimilate into mainstream school setting.

- Design visual aids that support child's needs
  Always ask for permission from teacher before

- introducing new materials*

- Guide child to accomplish goals in the following domains:

  1. Classroom routines and behaviors

  2. Social interaction with classmates

  3. Compliance with teacher's instructions

For school shadow support, you are working with *teachers*, *parents*, and *other educators* (e.g., *allied educators*). It is crucial to ensure that everyone is on the same page, working towards common goals for the child. Teachers have overall authority in the teaching of the class.

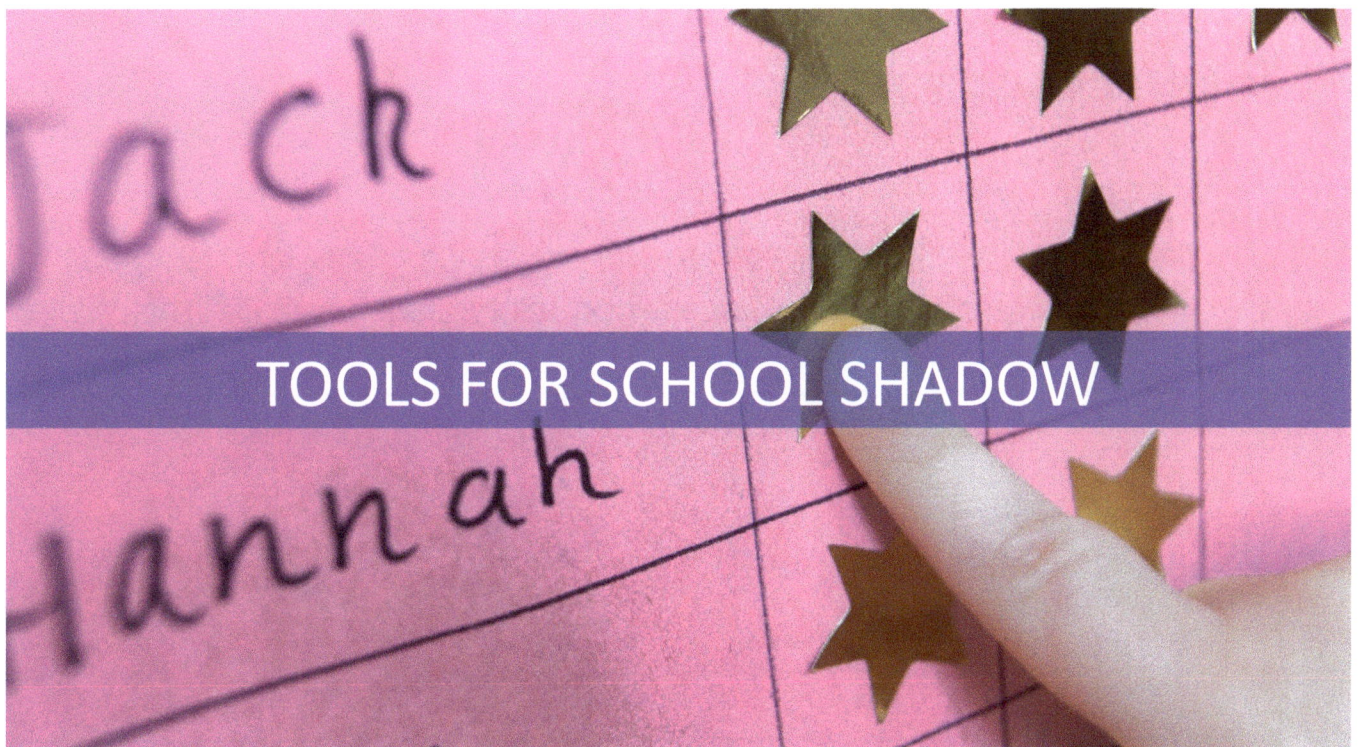

TOOLS FOR SCHOOL SHADOW

TOOLS FOR SCHOOL SHADOW

→ **The tools used for school shadow are generally around the same as the tools used for small group intervention.**

→ **However, at this stage, the shadow teacher has to coordinate with class teachers (e.g., find out timetable for the day) and ensure that implementation of the tools causes minimal disruption in the class.**

⋯→ *Token Economy*

PRESCHOOL

- For preschoolers, token economies typically look like this.

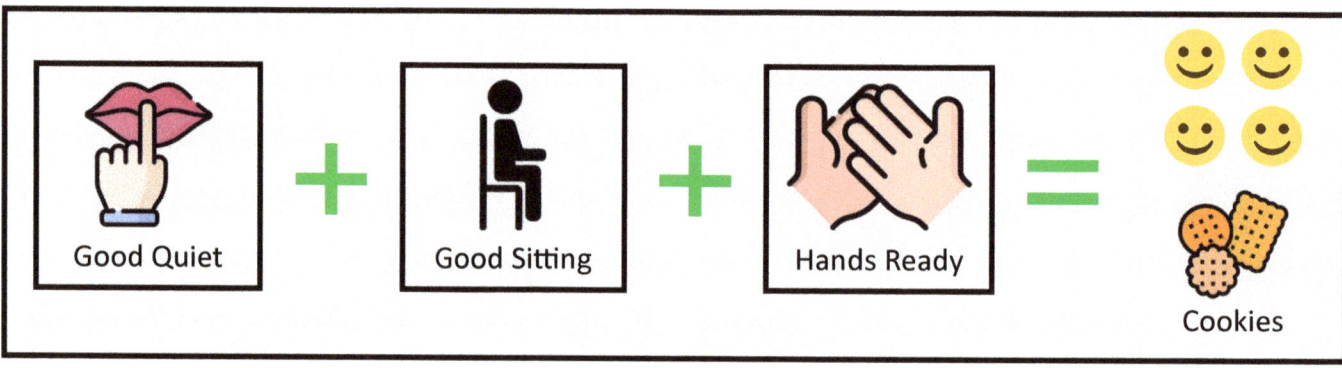

- Details on how to use the token economy can be found on page 18.

- Goals for the token economy must be adjusted and chosen based on the child (E.g., If the child faces difficulties sitting on the floor, a goal can be to sit on the floor, and the child earns a token whenever he sits on the floor nicely.).

- Reward can be stickers. If food is used, the shadow should give the food discreetly or during transitions so as to not disturb the other students.

···→ *Token Economy (continued)*

PRIMARY SCHOOL

- For primary school children, a more advanced token economy can be used.

Example:

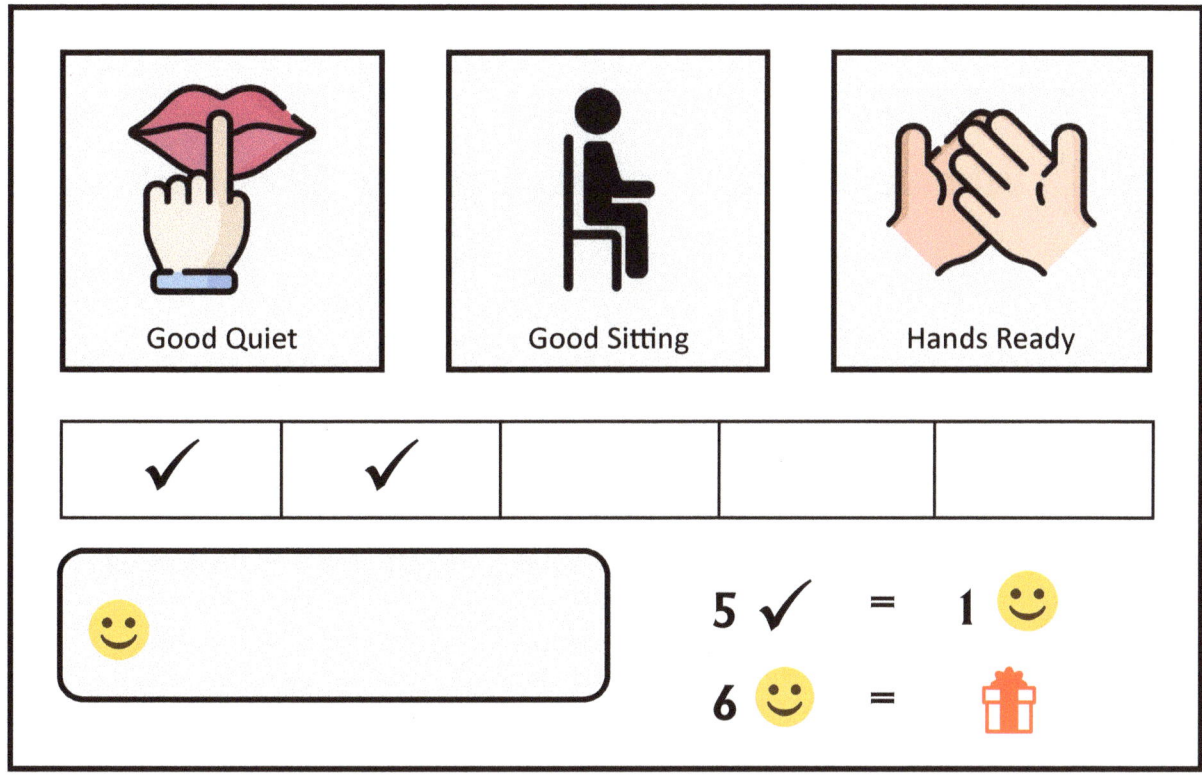

- However, if child is not ready to use the advanced version, shadow can choose to start from the basic preschool version and slowly progress to the more advanced one.

- Rewards must be desirable to the child and kept exclusive for school shadow to achieve maximum effectiveness.

⋯→ *Token Economy (continued)*

PRIMARY SCHOOL (continued)

How can I use the token economy?

(1) **At the start of the day, shadow chooses 3 goals**

(2) **Whenever child achieves a goal, a checkmark is given.**

(3) **Once 5 checkmarks are earned, child gets a smiley sticker. Checkmarks are then erased and restarted.**

(4) **Once child earns 6 stickers, child gets a reward.**

The number of checkmarks and stickers needed can be changed accordingly. For this token economy, child is constantly reinforced throughout the day and earns the reward at the end of the day.

⋯→ *Schedule*

PRESCHOOL

How can I use the schedule?

1 **The therapist prepares a schedule board with a variety of tasks that the child typically completes in school.**

Example:

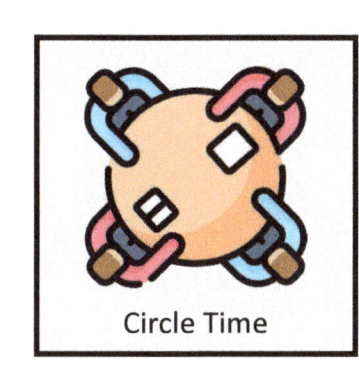
Circle Time

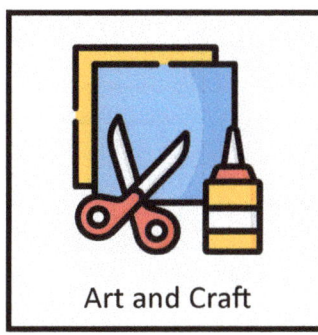
Art and Craft

Doing Writing

2 **At the start of the day, the therapist checks with the class teacher about the activities for the day and arranges the tasks on the schedule board.**

···→ *Schedule*

PRESCHOOL (continued)

How can I use the schedule?

3 Child checks off task or removes task from the board once it is completed.

4 Child moves on to the next task on the list till the end of the day.

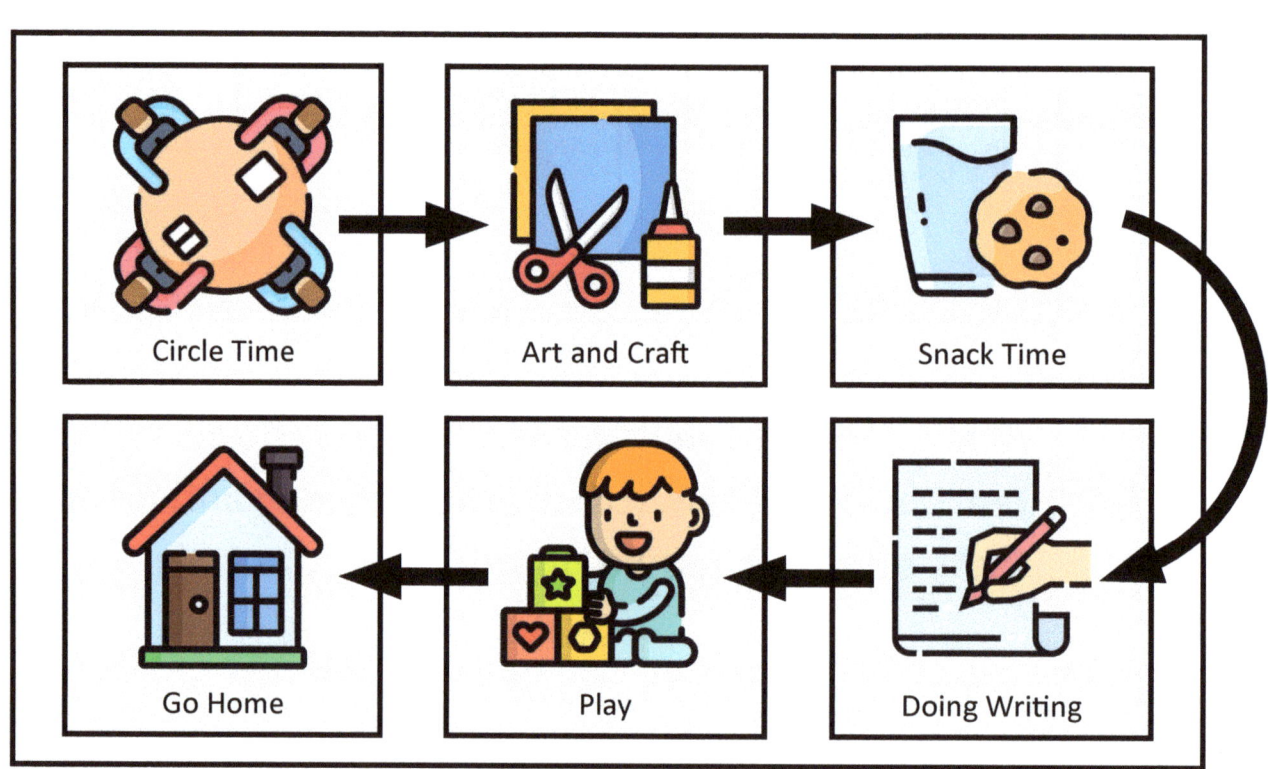

┈→ *Schedule*

PRIMARY SCHOOL

For primary school, the schedule is the class timetable. Some tips for timetable are as follows:

→ Timetable should be color-coded (one color for one subject that correspond to the file color for the subject).

→ Timetable should be small such that it does not take up too much space on the table.

→ Timetable can be either weekly or daily.

How to use a timetable

1 **Therapist prepares a color-coded timetable for the child and pastes it on the child's table**

2 **Therapist goes through the timetable for the day with the child at the start of the day.**

3 **The child checks off or cancels the subject after the class is over.**

⋯→ *Schedule (continued)*

PRIMARY SCHOOL (continued)

Weekly Timetable – Timetable for the entire week.

Times	MON	TUE	WED	THURS	FRI
07:40 – 08:10	EL	SS	EL	MT	EL
08:10 – 08:40	EL	SS	EL	MT	EL
08:40 – 09:10	EL	MT	EL	MT	MA
09:10 – 09:40	MA	MT	MA	ART	MA
09:40 – 10:10	MA	MT	MA	ART	MA
10:10 – 10:40	LUNCH				
10:40 – 11:05	PE	MA	EL	MA	MA
11:05 – 11:35	EL	MA	MT	MA	MA
11:35 – 12:05	EL	EL	MT	EL	EL
12:05 – 12:15	BREAK				
12:15 – 12:45	MT	EL	MU	EL	MU
12:45 – 1:15	MT	EL	MU	EL	PE
1:15 – 1:45	MT	PE	EL	EL	PE

⋯→ *Schedule (continued)*

PRIMARY SCHOOL (continued)

Daily Timetable – Timetable for the day. Shadow pastes the child's timetable for the day on child's table at the start of the day.

Monday									
08:00 – 08:30	08:30 – 09:00	09:00 – 09:30	09:30 – 10:00	10:00 – 10:30	10:30 – 11:00	11:00 – 11:30	11:30 – 12:00	12:00 – 12:30	12:00 – 01:00
EL	EL	MA	MA	LUNCH	MT	MT	MU	MU	PE

Tuesday									
08:00 – 08:30	08:30 – 09:00	09:00 – 09:30	09:30 – 10:00	10:00 – 10:30	10:30 – 11:00	11:00 – 11:30	11:30 – 12:00	12:00 – 12:30	12:00 – 01:00
MT	MT	EL	EL	LUNCH	ART	ART	ART	MA	MA

Wednesday									
08:00 – 08:30	08:30 – 09:00	09:00 – 09:30	09:30 – 10:00	10:00 – 10:30	10:30 – 11:00	11:00 – 11:30	11:30 – 12:00	12:00 – 12:30	12:00 – 01:00
MA	MA	SS	SS	LUNCH	MT	MT	EL	EL	MA

⋯→ *Routines*

Routines used for school shadow are similar to the ones used at home or during small group intervention. However, the steps have to be in accordance to the school's steps, and the pictures in the routine are real-life pictures of the school.

PRESCHOOL

Example 1: Morning routine

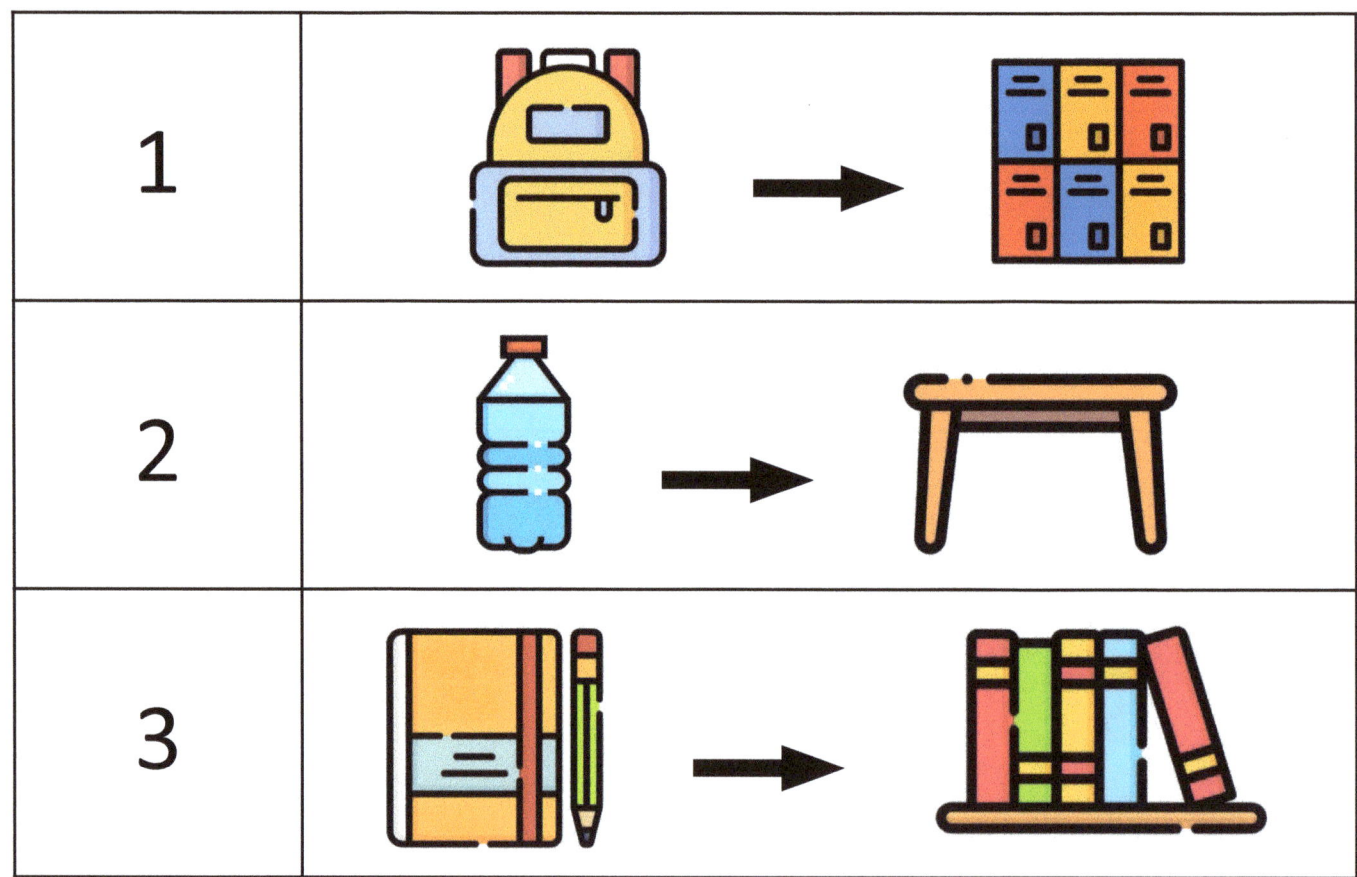

⋯→ *Routines*

PRESCHOOL (continued)

Example 2: Doing work routine

Goal: Build up good work habits

1	Take **pencil** and **eraser**
2	Write **name** and **date** **Name**: John Tan **Date**: _____
3	Do **worksheet**
4	Give to **teacher**
5	Keep **pencil** and **eraser**

⤍ *Routines*

PRESCHOOL (continued)

Example 3: Snack routine

1	Take **bottle**
2	Sit on **chair**
3	**Eat**
4	Clear **plate**

⋯→ *Routines*

PRIMARY SCHOOL

Example 1: Morning assembly routine

1	Stand in attention
2	Sing national anthem
3	Take pledge
4	Sit down
5	Listen to teacher

···→ **Routines**

PRIMARY SCHOOL

Example 2: Meal routine

1	Think of what to buy
2	Line up
3	Order my food Can I have _____ please?
4	Pay money
5	Take change
6	Sit at table and eat

⸻➤ *Visuals*

PRIMARY SCHOOL

Visuals are used to prompt the child of appropriate behaviors in a classroom setting. With visual prompts, child will be less reliant on verbal prompts, making it easier for eventual fading of shadow.

How can I use visuals?

Therapist prepares a color-coded timetable for the child and pastes it on the child's table

1 **When child needs behavioral prompts, show child appropriate visual card**

(E.g., child verbal stimming ➜ show child quiet mouth card)

2 **If child displays good behaviors, praise!**

3 **If child does not respond to visuals, gently tap child and redirect to visual.**

⤍ *Visuals*

Here are some common visuals:

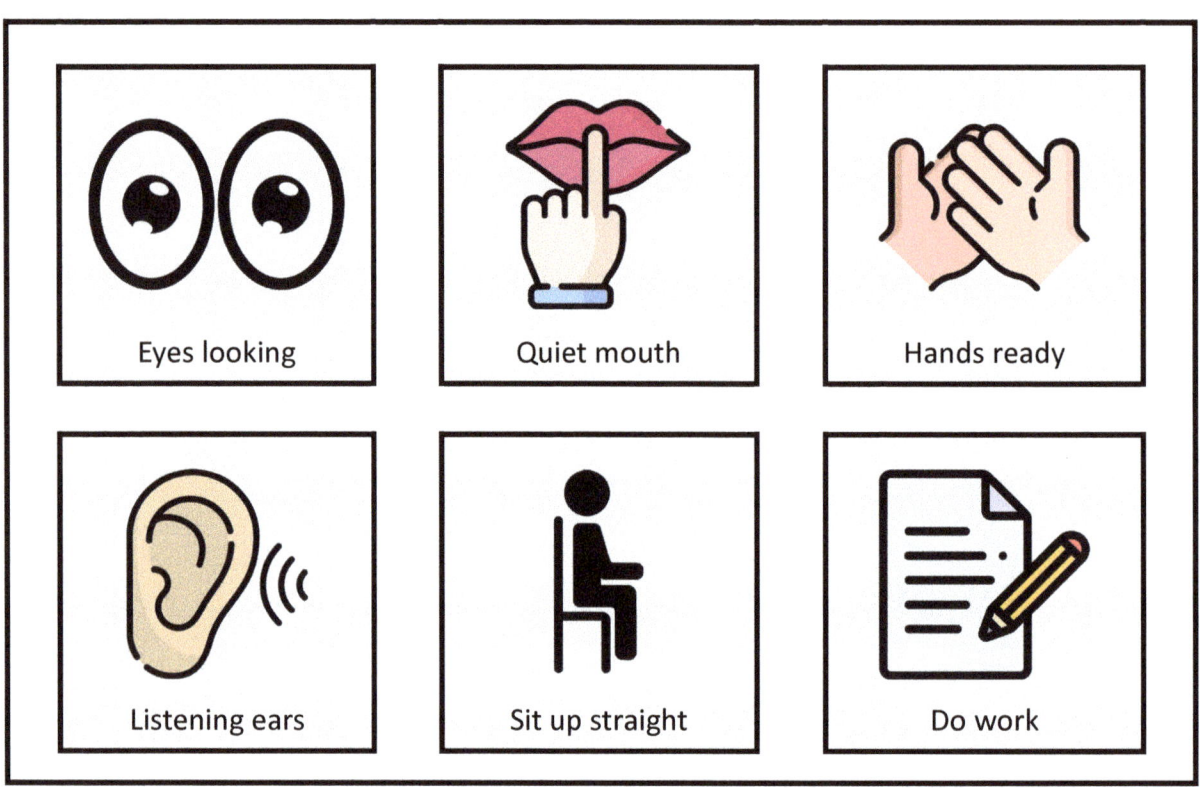

Create other visuals based on child's needs!

···→ *Social story*

Social stories help teach children appropriate social behaviors in a story form. Whenever the shadow teacher sees a challenge faced by the child, the shadow teacher can create a social story based on the situation.

Social stories should be:

(1) **Visual-based**

➜ Social stories should include many pictures.

➜ As much as possible, these pictures should be real-life pictures.

(2) **Positive**

➜ Positive statements should be used (e.g., I can keep calm).

➜ Negative statements should be avoided (e.g., I do not get angry).

(3) **At child's language ability levels**

➜ Language should not be too difficult for the child.

➜ Child must be able to understand the language used.

⤳ *Social story*

Example 1:

CIRCLE TIME

My name is John. 🧑 **In school** 🏫 **, I have circle time!** 🔵 **During circle time, I listen,** 👂 **keep quiet,** 🤫 **and cross my legs.** 🧘 **If I want to say something, I raise my hand.** 🙋

⋯→ *Social story*

Example 2:

PLAYING WITH FRIENDS

My name is John. In school I have many

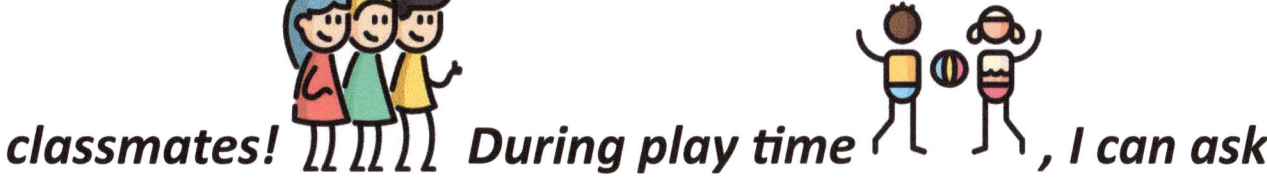

classmates! During play time , I can ask

my friends to play together! Can I play with you? If my friend

says "No," it's okay! I can play with another

friend!

⋯→ *Check-In & Check-Out*

(For primary school children only)

Check-in & check-out works as a reward chart, meaning the child gets reinforced after the end of every lesson if he reaches predetermined goals.

How can I use check-in & check-out?

1 **Set goals and explain the goals to the child.**

2 **At the end of each lesson, give a checkmark to the child if the child achieves all the goals.**

3 **At the end of the week, child earns the reward (if any) according to the number of checkmarks earned.**

⋯→ *Check-In & Check-Out*

(For primary school children only)

Example of check-in & check-out

Check-in & check-out for Adam				
Mon	**Tue**	**Wed**	**Thurs**	**Fri**
EL	PE	MT	MT	EL
MA	EL	MA	EL	MT
MT	MT	EL	MA	MA
ART	MU	SS	PE	SS

Earn a checkmark for each
period if 3 criterions are met:

1. No hitting friends

2. Do all my work

3. No walking around
   the class

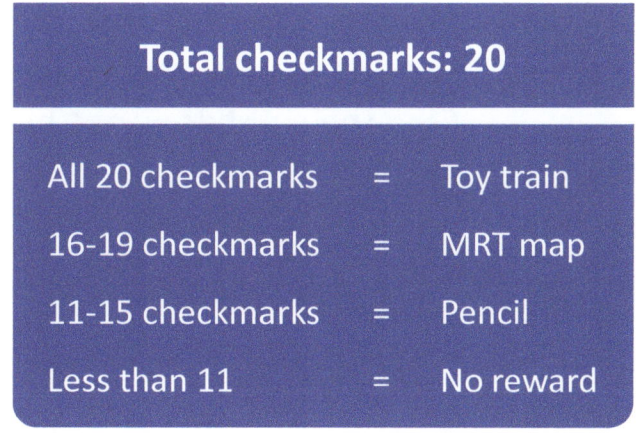

Total checkmarks: 20

All 20 checkmarks	=	Toy train
16-19 checkmarks	=	MRT map
11-15 checkmarks	=	Pencil
Less than 11	=	No reward

⋯→ *Behavioral Contracts*
(For primary school children only)

Behavioral contracts are useful, especially when a child consistently has issues in one area (e.g., hitting other students in the class).

How can I use a behavioral contract?

1 **Set up the goal and explain the behavioral contract to the child**

E.g., "If you keep your hands to yourself and don't hit anyone for the entire day, you will get a signature from me at the end of the day. If you get all the signatures, you get a surprise reward!"

2 **If the child reaches the goal, the shadow and child sign the contract at the end of the day.**

E.g., the child does not hit anyone for the entire day.

→ Making the child sign the contract gives him a sense of ownership to what is agreed upon, hence making him more likely to succeed.

3 **At the end of the week, if child earns a signature for all 5 days, the child gets the reward.**

···→ *Behavioral Contracts*

(For primary school children only)

Example of behavioral contract

NO HITTING

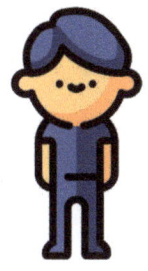
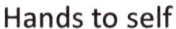

Hands to self

Do not hit

For the week from: **7/30 – 8/3**

Please sign beside your name after each day if Ms. Tan
is satisfied with your behavior.

Date	7/30	7/31	8/1	8/2	8/3
ADAM					
MS. TAN					

If I manage to earn **ALL** signatures, I will get a **toy train*** from Ms .Tan!

_____   _____

Adam's Signature   Ms. Tan's Signature

---

* Reward can be decided by the child. Give child options of rewards which are deemed reasonable by parents/teachers.

Chapter 7

SOCIAL SKILLS DEVELOPMENT

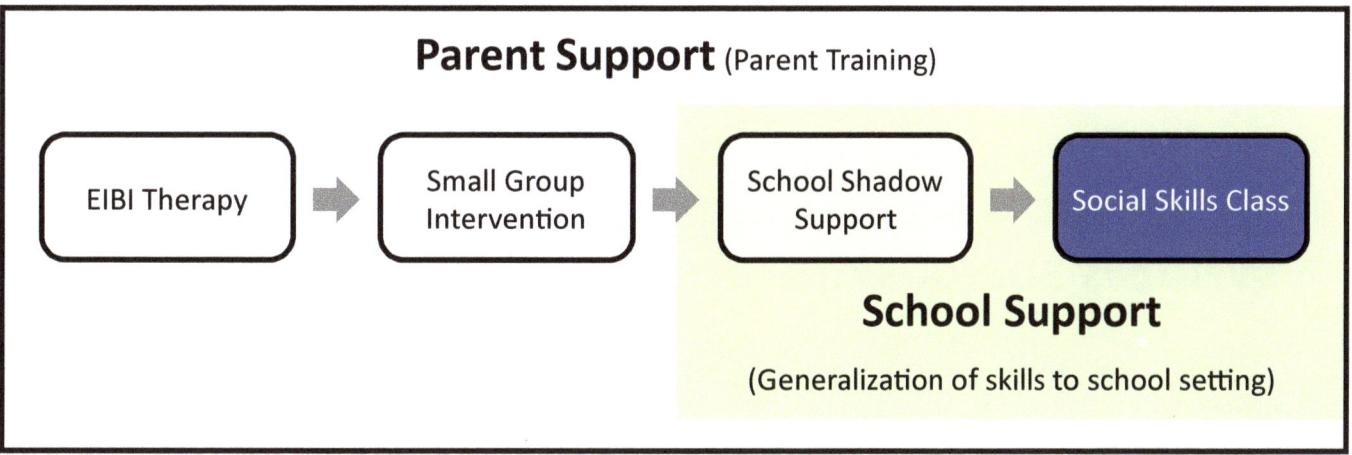

The next stage of the CMEI model is focused on social skills development. In this stage, the child learns more advanced social skills in a group setting.

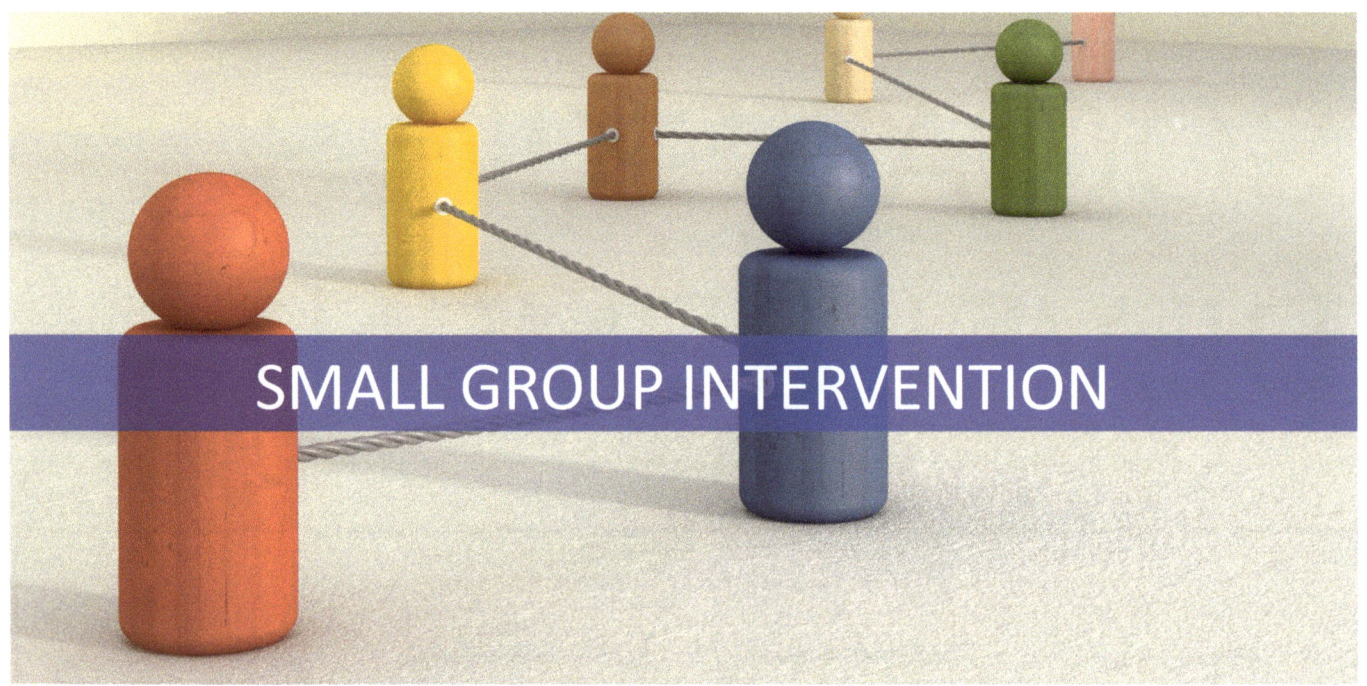

SMALL GROUP INTERVENTION

···→ *What is social skills development?*

Social skills development targets the development of skills such as recognizing facial expressions and body gestures, inferring from situations, and learning about social consequences and social dilemmas. In this chapter, two different levels of social skills are introduced.

Social Skills (Foundation)

For children 4-10 years old with basic to good verbal and reading skills.

Social Skills (Advanced)

For children 7-13 years old with good verbal and reading skills.

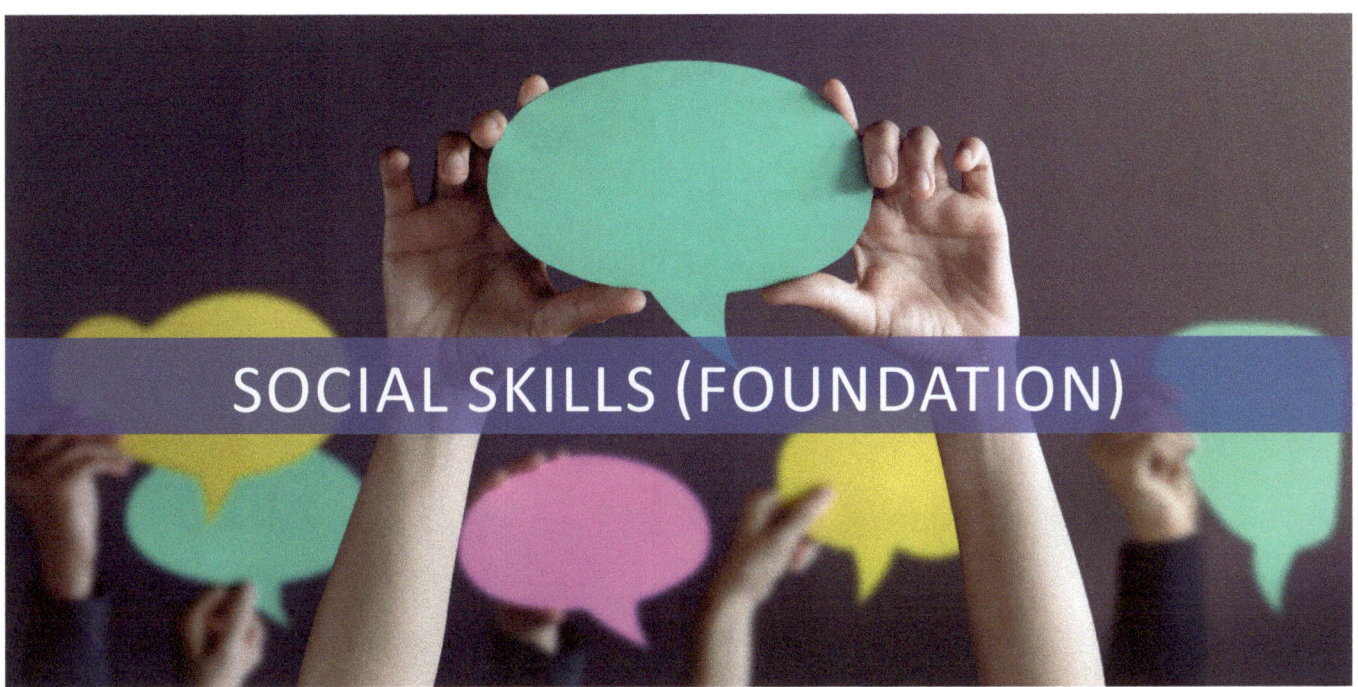

- The foundation social skills program focuses mainly on the fundamental socio-cognitive skills and language skills needed to navigate social interaction.

- Primary skill objectives (e.g., awareness of self, emotions) are addressed while recurring secondary skills are practiced throughout the entire program.

- Some of the recurring secondary skills include: turn- taking, joint attention, creative-thinking, auditory comprehension, verbal and non-verbal expressions, sharing, joining in, and teamwork.

SOCIAL SKILLS (FOUNDATION)

⋯→ *Target audience*

- For children ages 4-10 with basic to good verbal and reading skills

With Fundamental Skills Deficits, Such As:

❑ Difficulties regulating non-verbal behaviors such as eye contact, facial expressions, and body postures

❑ Atypical prosody of speech such as speaking in a flat and monotonous voice

❑ Difficulties with inferring people's emotional states from facial, body and situation cues

❑ Difficulties with identifying and reciprocating to others' perspectives and emotions

❑ Issues in comprehending verbal responses

❑ Issues in deductive reasoning and in problem-solving to produce appropriate replies

⋯→ *Examples of tasks*

INTRODUCING YOURSELF

1. Write steps for introducing self when meeting someone new on the whiteboard

   > 1. Stand up
   >
   > 2. Look at the other person in the eye
   >
   > 3. Smile
   >
   > 4. Say "Hi, I am _____."

2. Children roleplay with each other using the steps, taking turns to introduce themselves to each other.

Adapted from *101 Ways to Teach Children Social Skills* by Lawrence E. Shapiro (2004)

···→ *Examples of tasks*

LEARNING ABOUT SELF AND OTHERS

1. Tell the group that different people have different interests, though some interests may be repeated.

Color	Activities	Food
Song	Places	School subjects

2. On the whiteboard, write the following:

3. Children take turns to tell one of their favorite things under each category. Teacher writes each thing down on whiteboard under the heading.

4. Reinforce the idea that some children may have similar interests, and others have unique interests.

Adapted from *101 Ways to Teach Children Social Skills* by Lawrence E. Shapiro (2004)

⟶ *Examples of tasks*

FACIAL EXPRESSIONS

1. Print out pictures with different facial expressions

2. For each picture, ask child:

   → What is the facial expression saying?

   → Why do you think the person feels that way?

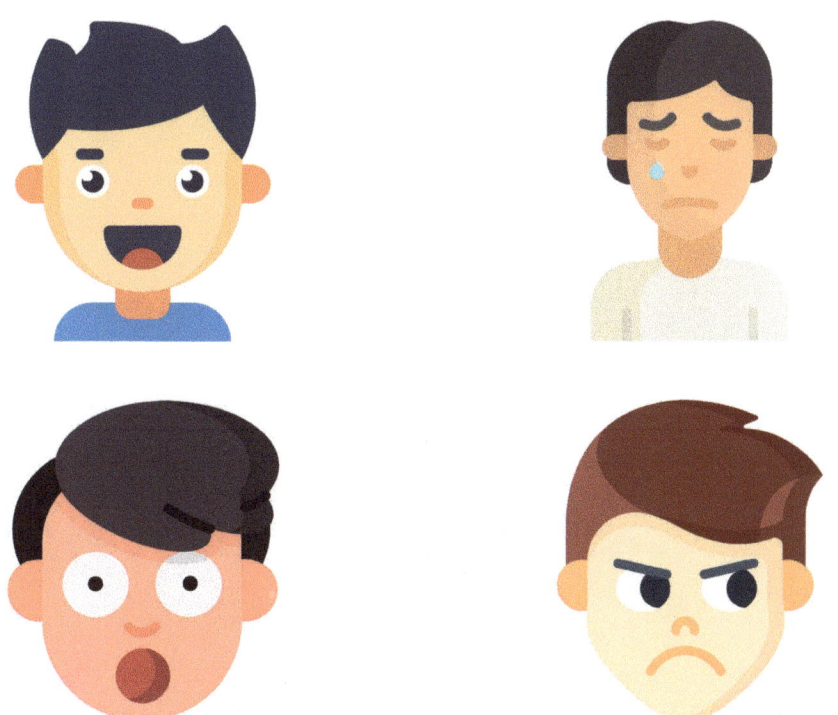

Adapted from *101 Ways to Teach Children Social Skills* by Lawrence E. Shapiro (2004)

⋯→ *Examples of tasks*

BODY GESTURES

1. Print out pictures with different gestures.

2. For each picture, ask the child:

   → What does this gesture mean?

   → Describe a time this gesture might be used.

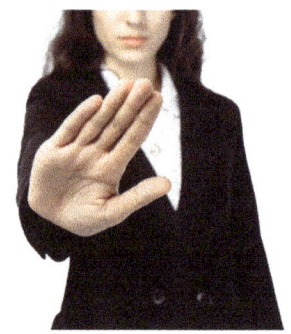
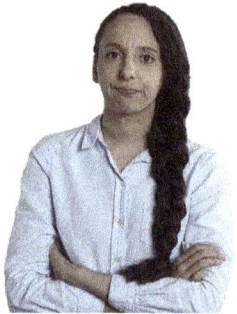
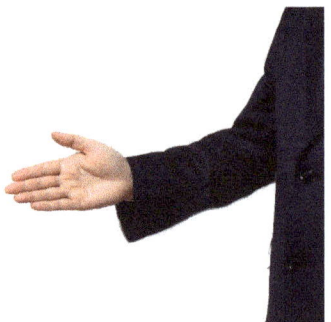
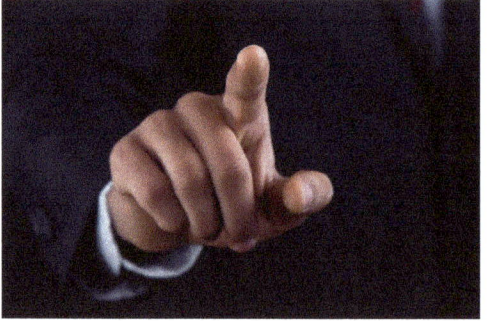

Adapted from *101 Ways to Teach Children Social Skills* by Lawrence E. Shapiro (2004)

···→ *Examples of tasks*

VOICE VOLUME

1. Explain to the children the importance of the right volume of voice in different situations.

2. Hand the children a worksheet with different scenarios and get them to checkmark the voice volume that is appropriate for that situation.

	SOFT	NORMAL	LOUD
1. In a library			
2. At a basketball game			
3. Playing outdoors			
4. Playing indoors			
5. When someone is sleeping			
6. Watching a movie			
7. Shopping at a store			

Adapted from *101 Ways to Teach Children Social Skills* by Lawrence E. Shapiro (2004)

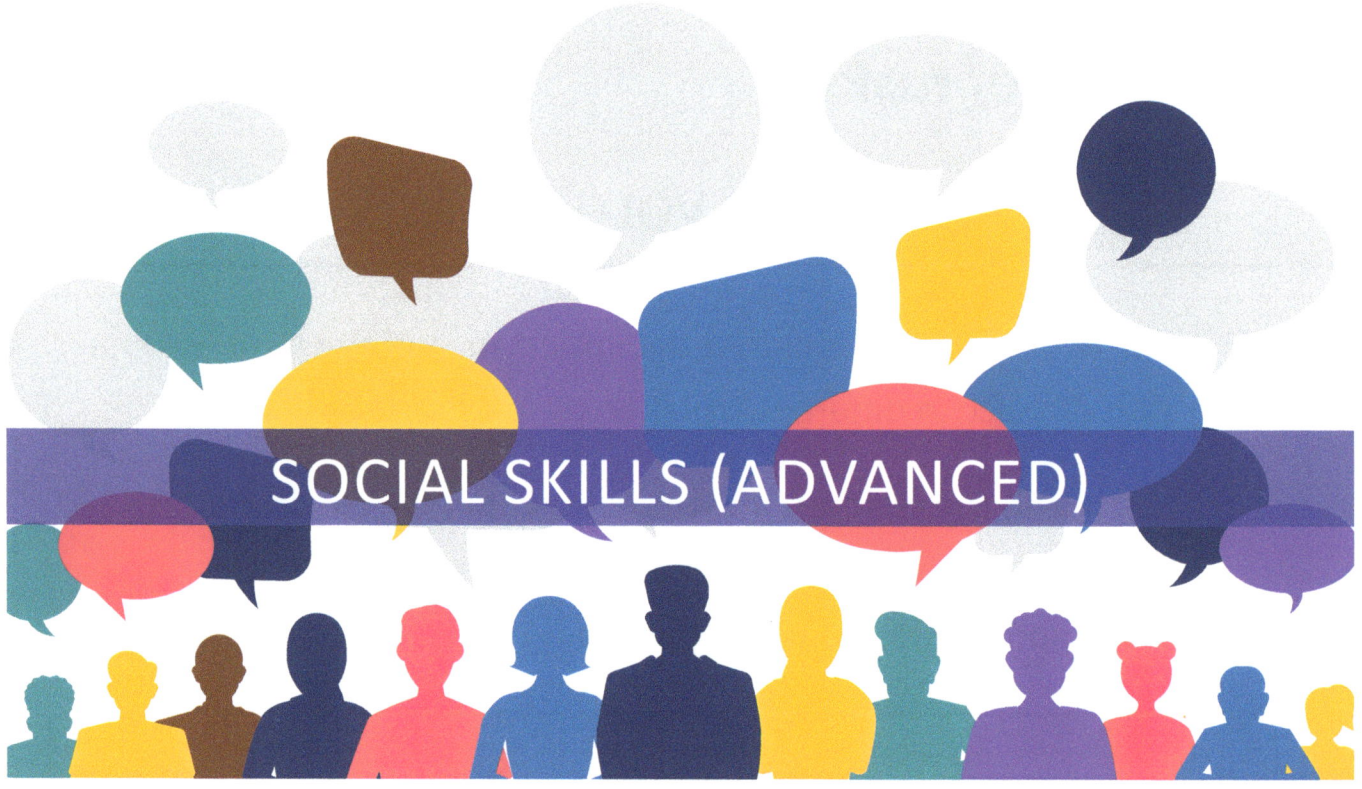

- The advanced social skills program has a deeper focus on conversation techniques. More advanced conversation skills such as asking for favors, negotiating, offering advices, and rationalizing criticisms will be practiced.

- Complex social situations will be introduced in the curriculum. The programs involve deeper discussions, as situations touched on may not have clear-cut right or wrong answers.

- Similarly, primary skill objectives (e.g., complex emotions) are addressed while recurring secondary skills will be practiced throughout the entire program.

SOCIAL SKILLS (ADVANCED)

⋯→ *Target audience*

- For children ages 7-13 with good verbal and reading skills

With Fundamental Skills Deficits, Such As:

❑ Issues with deductive reasoning and problem solving to produce appropriate replies

❑ Issues with conversing with others

❑ Issues with making and maintaining friendship

❑ Rationalizing criticism and making good decisions

❑ Empathizing with others

⸱⸱⸱➔ *Examples of tasks*

CONSEQUENCES

1. Therapist describes a situation to the children.

2. Therapist comes up with 3 options to handle the situation together with the child.

3. Children discuss consequence for each option.

4. Children take a vote on the best option based on the consequences.

SITUATION: FRIEND DOES NOT WANT TO PLAY WITH ME

	Option	Consequence
1		
2		
3		

BEST OPTION: _____

⋯→ *Examples of tasks*

KINDNESS

1. Print out cards with different pictures/description of actions.

Lending my friend my eraser when he forgets to bring his	**Laughing at my friend when he falls**	**Taking care of my friend when he is sick**

2. Children take turns to pick an action, read out the action to the class, and tell the class if it is a kind action or not.

3. Whenever child displays kind actions, therapist reinforces child (e.g., by praising child in front of class and explaining to class that child's action was kind).

···→ *Examples of tasks*

ASKING QUESTIONS

1. Therapist explains to the children the importance of asking relevant questions to keep conversations going.

2. Therapist practices with the children by coming up with a few sentences and getting the children to take turns asking a question related to the sentence.

Therapist	Child
I have a dog	What is his name?
Dusty	What kind of dog is he?
A golden retriever	

3. Therapist continues answering the children's questions and sees how many questions the children can continue to ask!

Adapted from *101 Ways to Teach Children Social Skills* by Lawrence E. Shapiro (2004)

⋯→ *Examples of tasks*

EXPRESSING THEMSELVES

The therapist can guide the child in expressing their feelings through roleplay by following these steps:

1. Say how you feel ("I feel…")

2. Tell the other person what they did that made you feel that way ("when you…")

3. Describe how you were affected ("because…")

4. State what would make the situation better for you ("and I want…)

---

1. I feel **happy** when you _____ because _____ and I want _____ .

2. I feel **frustrated** when you _____ because _____ and I want _____ .

3. I feel _____ when you _____ because _____ and I want _____ .

Adapted from *101 Ways to Teach Children Social Skills* by Lawrence E. Shapiro (2004)

⋯→ *Examples of tasks*

MIXED EMOTIONS

1. Therapist explains to the children that many times, we feel more than one emotion.

2. Therapist goes through with children different scenarios and get them to identify two or more emotions that the person may be feeling.

It is my first day at school.

"I feel _____ but I also feel _____."

I got a present for my birthday but it wasn't what I was hoping for.

"I feel _____ but I also feel _____."

My mother accidently broke my favourite toy but is going to buy me a new one.

"I feel _____ but I also feel _____."

Adapted from *101 Ways to Teach Children Social Skills* by Lawrence E. Shapiro (2004)

Chapter 8

PARENT SUPPORT

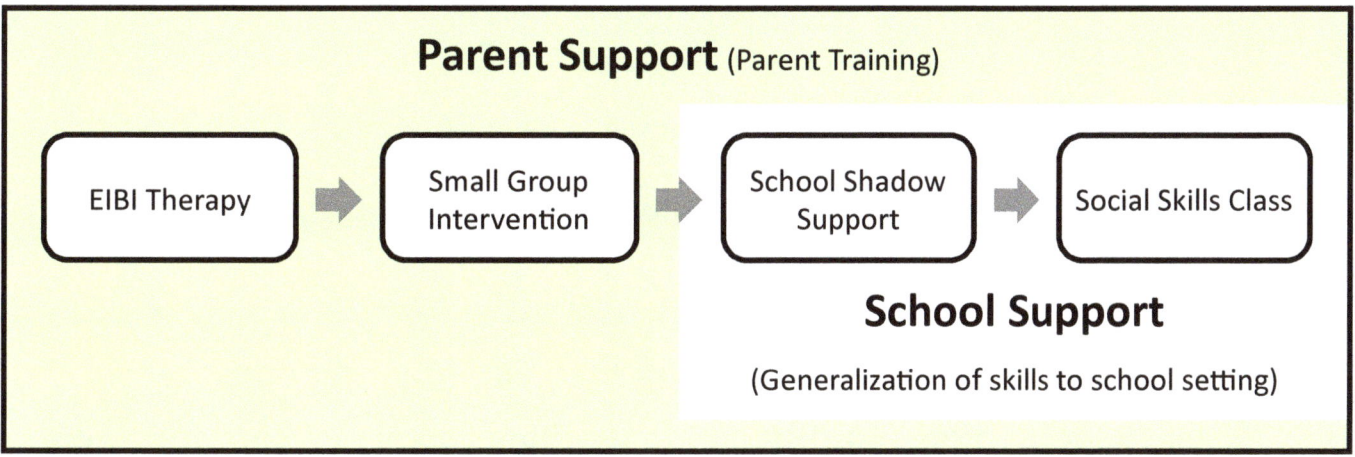

Parent Support (Parent Training)

| EIBI Therapy | → | Small Group Intervention | → | School Shadow Support | → | Social Skills Class |

School Support

(Generalization of skills to school setting)

Through all the stages of CMEI, parents play a crucial role. It is important that parents are involved in the child's intervention and development to help the child learn faster.

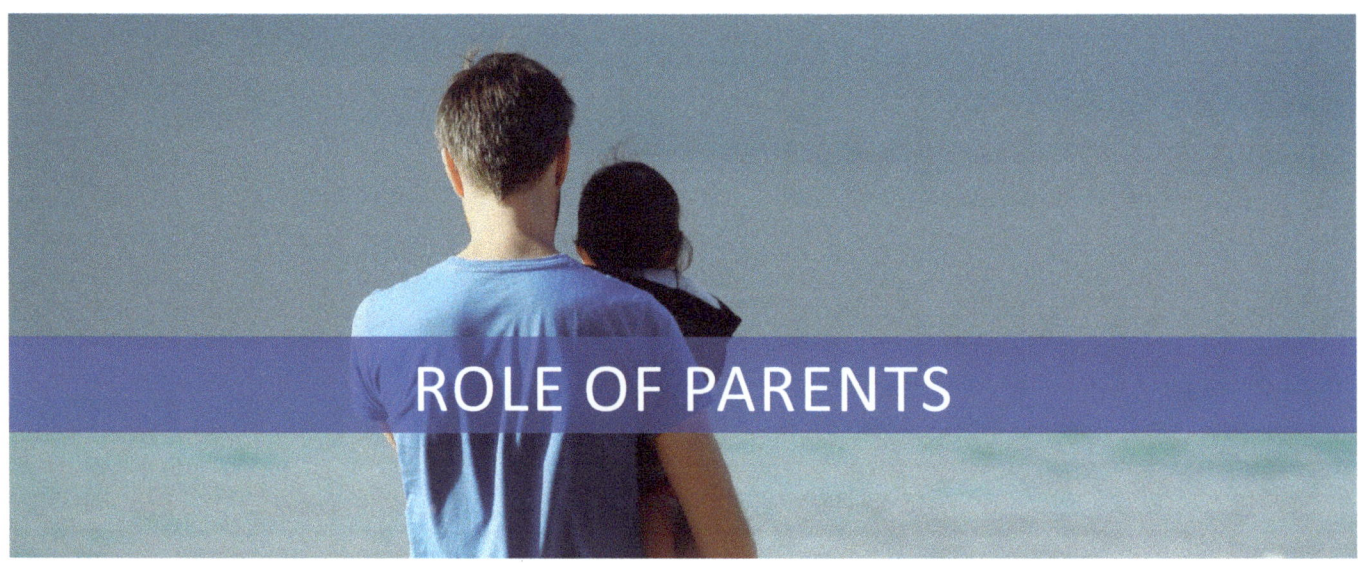

ROLE OF PARENTS

Parents can:

→ **Ensure that child receives timely and suitable intervention in the different phases**

→ **Work with all individuals helping the child (e.g., therapists, teachers) and ensure that all are working towards a common goal**

→ **Generalize what child learned during sessions in daily home settings in order to help child progress faster.**

→ **Follow up with child on intervention (e.g., reading social stories to child daily, having a token economy system at home)**

→ **Work with child regularly (recommended at least 2-3 times per week) to build the child's compliance at home**

→ **Change environment in the house to better suit the needs of child (Chapter 2)**

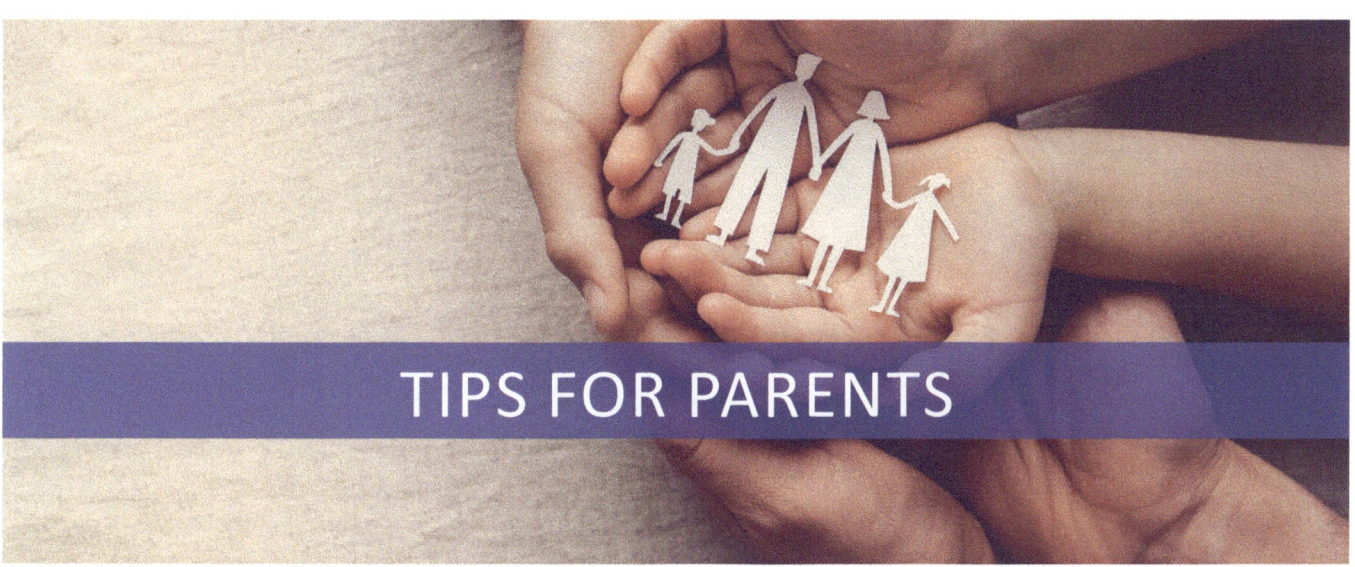

→ **Parents can start with baby steps. For a start, parents can work one-on-one with child with a schedule of 2 to 3 tasks. After building up the child's confidence, parents can increase the number of tasks and work cycles with the child.**

→ **Parents should see little improvements as achievements.**

→ **Parents should expect good and bad days.**

→ **Both parents must take a proactive approach in working with the child instead of relying only on one parent.**

→ **When in doubt, parents should seek advice from therapists.**

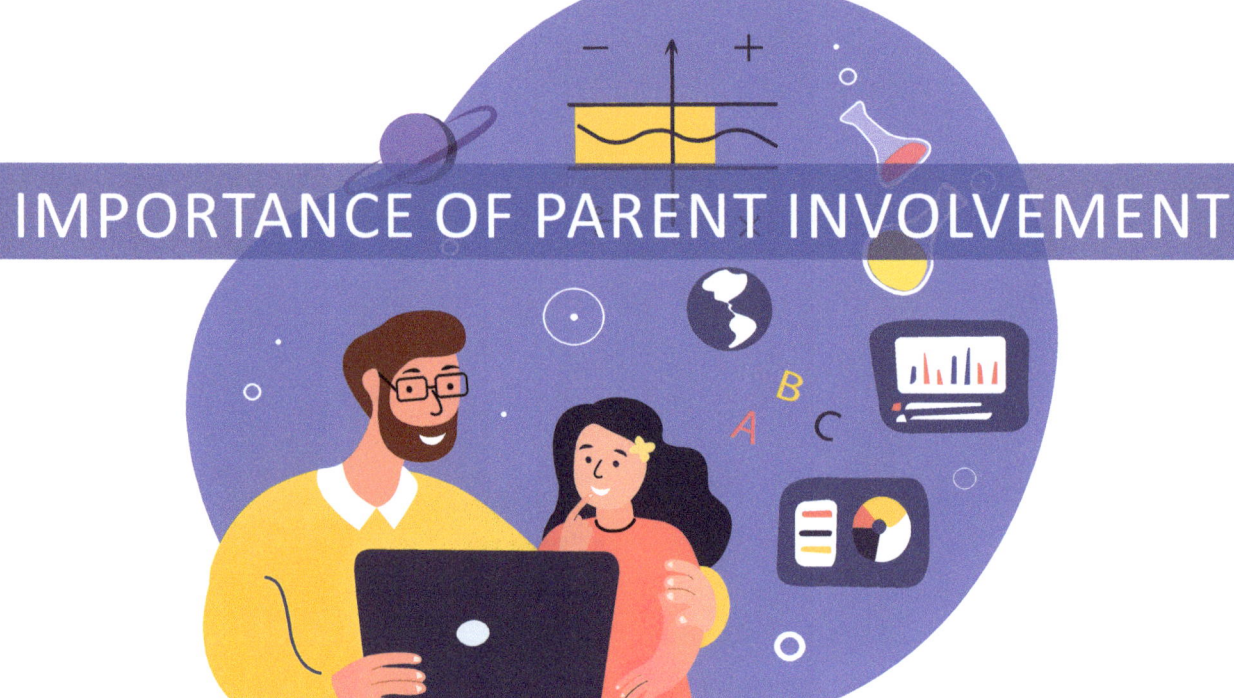

IMPORTANCE OF PARENT INVOLVEMENT

Parents, indeed, play a very important role in their child's development, as seen by the large research supporting the involvement of parents. Examples include:

→ Parental involvement improves generalizability of skills (Burrell & Burrego, 2011)

→ Parents who worked with children with autism from a young age helped reduce the severity of their symptoms and helps improve communication (Pickles et al., 2016)

→ Parents who received training changed the way they communicate and interact with the child, which leads to improving child communication and mitigating symptoms of autism (Senthilingam, 2016)

Chapter 9

CONTINGENCY PLANS

It is important for parents to prepare for situations that may happen so they will be able to respond appropriately in the best way when met with the situation. In this chapter, contingency plans for four situations that commonly happen with children with autism will be discussed.

1. **Handling meltdowns**

2. **Handling hitting/biting**

3. **Handling throwing**

4. **Handling screaming**

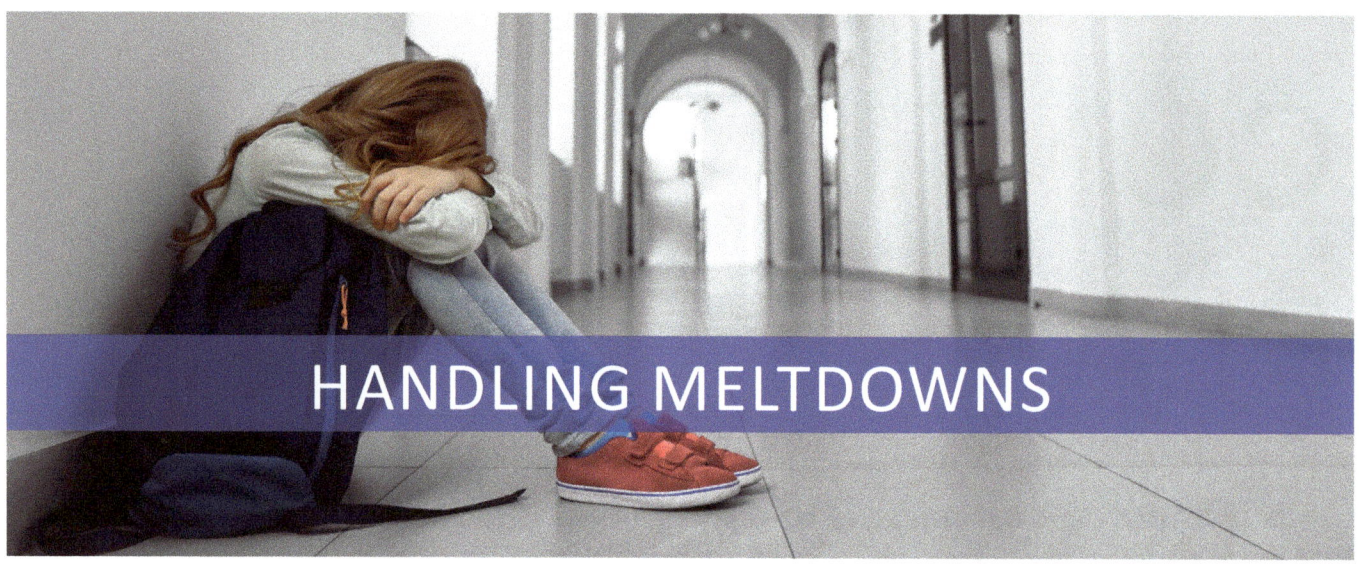

HANDLING MELTDOWNS

⋯→ *What is a meltdown?*

A meltdown is an intense reaction to an overwhelming situation. It is usually caused by the child having a sensory overload. The cause of meltdown differs for each child.

Common causes of meltdown include:

→ **Loud noises**

→ **Changes to routines**

→ **Intense emotions**

HANDLING MELTDOWNS

⋯→ *Tools for handling meltdowns*

Creating Calm Corner

A calm corner is a specific place in the house where a child can go to when a meltdown is escalating. Examples of places suitable to be a calm corner include a quiet room, the bed, or even just a chair.

Examples:

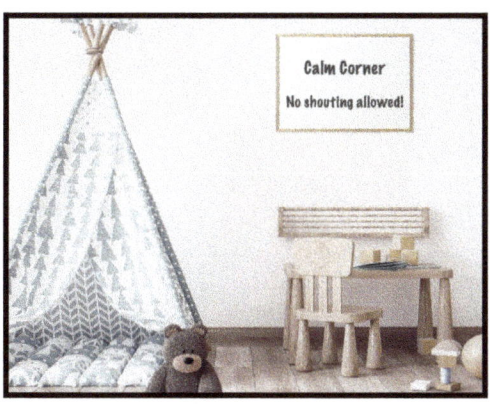
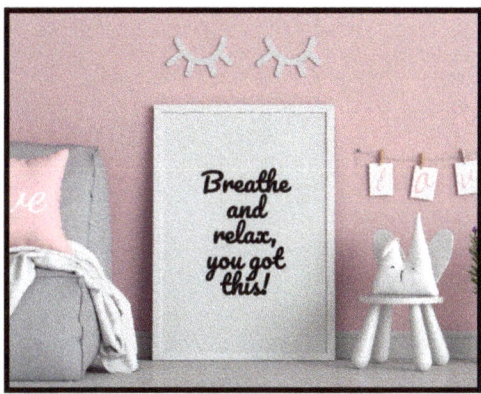

⟶ *Tools for handling meltdowns*

Calming Visual Routine

1	Take deep **breaths**	
2	Drink **water**	
3	Go to **calm corner**	
4	Set **timer** for 10 minutes	
5	Resume **normal** activities after time is up	

⤳ *Tools for handling meltdowns*

CREATE ANGER THERMOMETER

An anger thermometer helps the child understand their emotions and provides the child with solutions to manage their emotions.

Ben's Anger Thermometer

5	I am screaming and hitting myself	Go to calm corner for 5 minutes
4	I start hitting myself	I jump 10 times
3	I start talking loudly	I drink some water
2	I start to talk a lot	I take deep breaths
1	I feel calm!	Remain as is

The ways child displays anger at the different levels differs. Find out how your child displays their emotions!

Parents need to find ways that is effective for the child to calm down.

⇢ *Tools for handling meltdowns*

Create anger thermometer

How can I use an anger thermometer?

1 **Point out to child which level he is at**

E.g., "Look, Ben! You are starting to talk a lot! You are at level 2!"

2 **Ask child what he should do, while pointing at the corresponding actions for that level**

E.g., "What should you do when you are at level 2?"

3 **If child is unable to answer, let child know what he is supposed to do and do it with the child**

E.g. ,"Let's take deep breaths! 1, 2, 3, 4 ..."

4 **Praise child when he calms down**

E.g., "Wow! Good job calming down!"

⋯→ *What can I do during a meltdown?*

Ensure safety

→ Remove dangerous objects in surroundings

→ Move child away from hazardous objects

→ Monitor child closely until child calms down

→ Attempt to stop any behaviors that causes harm to self or others

Get child to follow calming routine

1	Take deep **breaths**	
2	Drink **water**	
3	Go to **calm corner**	
4	Set **timer** for 10 minutes	
5	Resume **normal** activities after time is up	

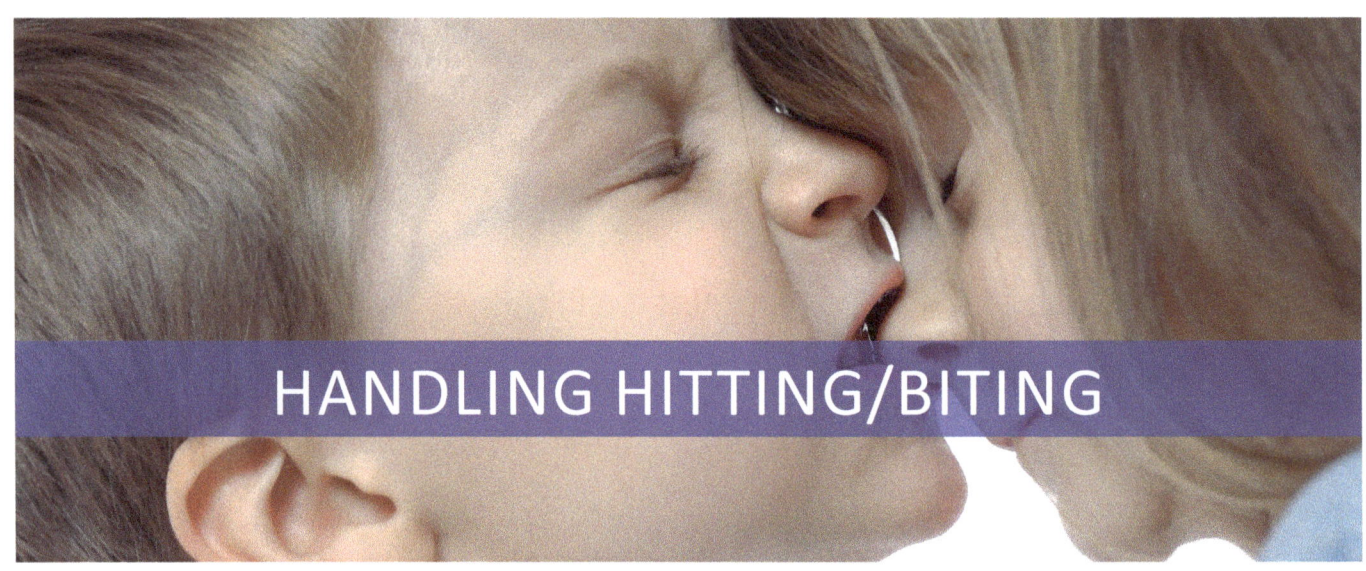

HANDLING HITTING/BITING

1 Tell child a firm "no" with no expressions

2 Timeout for around 1 minute until child is calm. Do NOT react until time is up.

3 Go back to task/activity. If hitting/biting was due to task, make task easier.

4 If it was a socially triggered situation, address the problem with social stories.

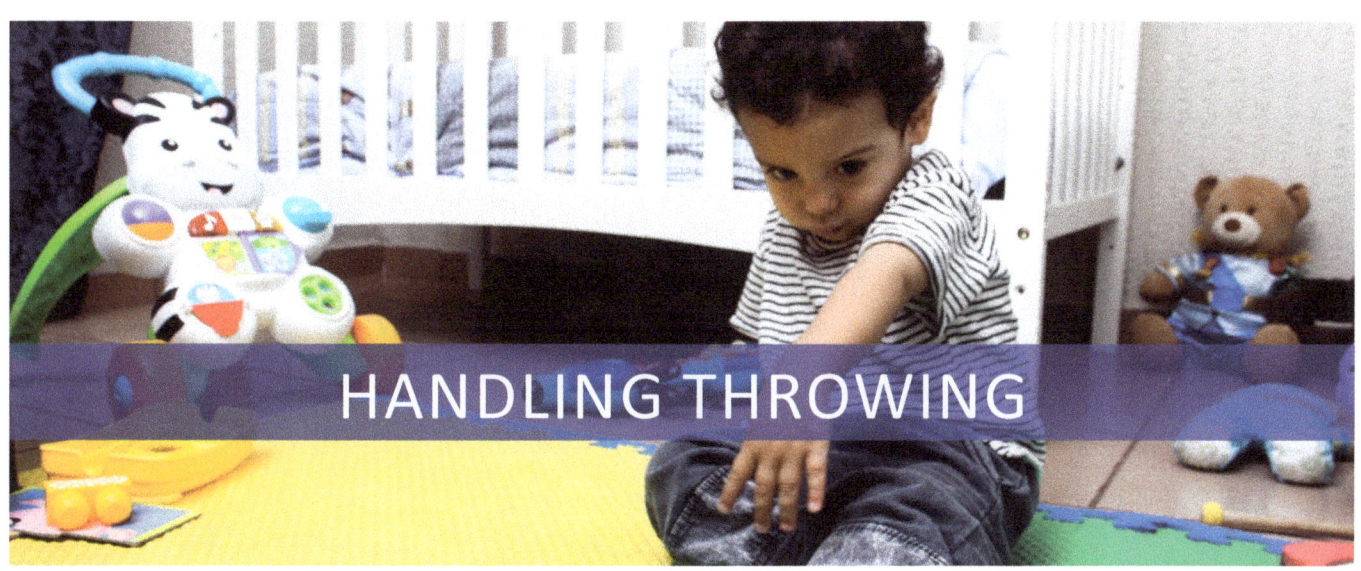

HANDLING THROWING

1 Tell child a firm "no" with no expressions

2 Use hand-over-hand to pick up toy (natural consequence)

3 Go back to task/activity.

4 If child continues task without throwing, praise the child!
If child throws again, repeat from step 1.

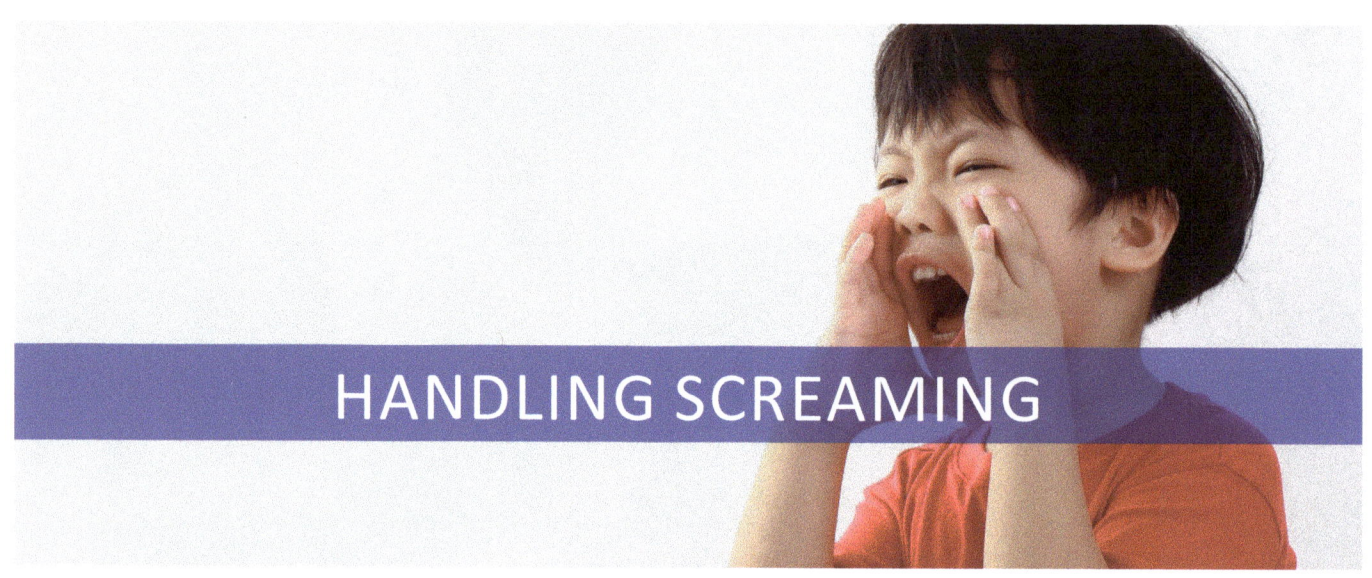

HANDLING SCREAMING

Screaming is often a sign of an escalating meltdown.

1 **Tell child a firm "no" with no expressions**

2 **Remove child from triggering stimulus**

3 **When child calms down, bring child back to where he was and resume normal activities**

4 **If he does well, praise!**

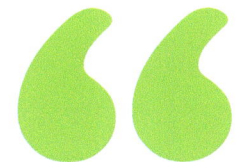

Every student can learn, just not the same day, or in the same way.

GEORGE EVANS

Chapter 10

TRANSITION TO PRIMARY ONE

Transitioning to a new school can be stressful for both the child and parents. Therefore, it is important to prepare early for a smoother transition.

In this final chapter, tools for a smoother transition will be introduced.

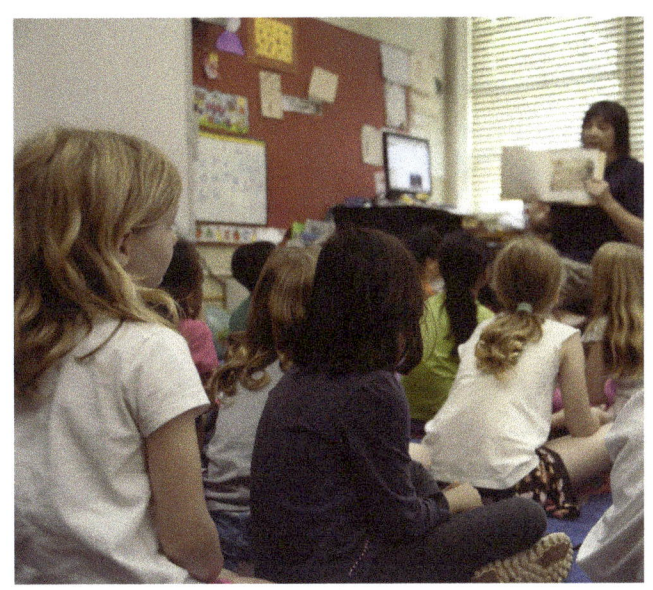

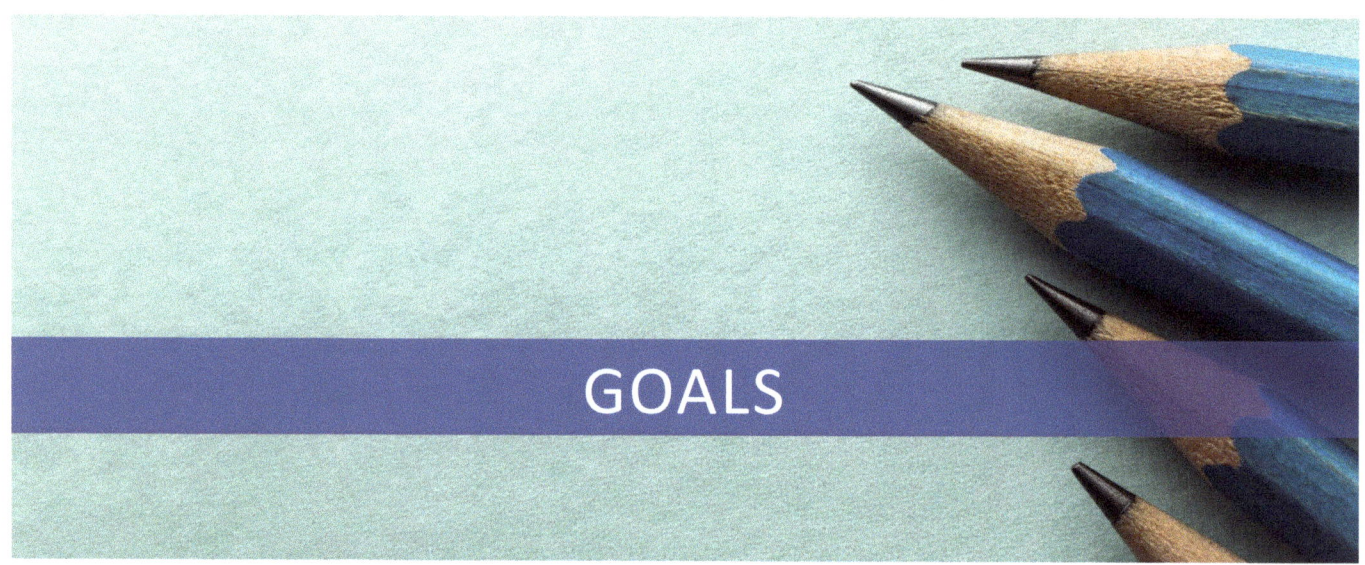

GOALS

Before the start of the school year, parents should arrange a meeting with school personnel (e.g., form teachers, subject teachers, allied educators). All individuals working with child must agree to a common set of goals to be reviewed monthly for the first 3 months. The goals can be revised only when the child is consistent in achieving all goals.

Initially, key goals include:

1. Compliance in class

2. Work habits

3. Adherence to school routines throughout the day

Once these goals are achieved, parents can focus on academic and social skills (Chapter 7).

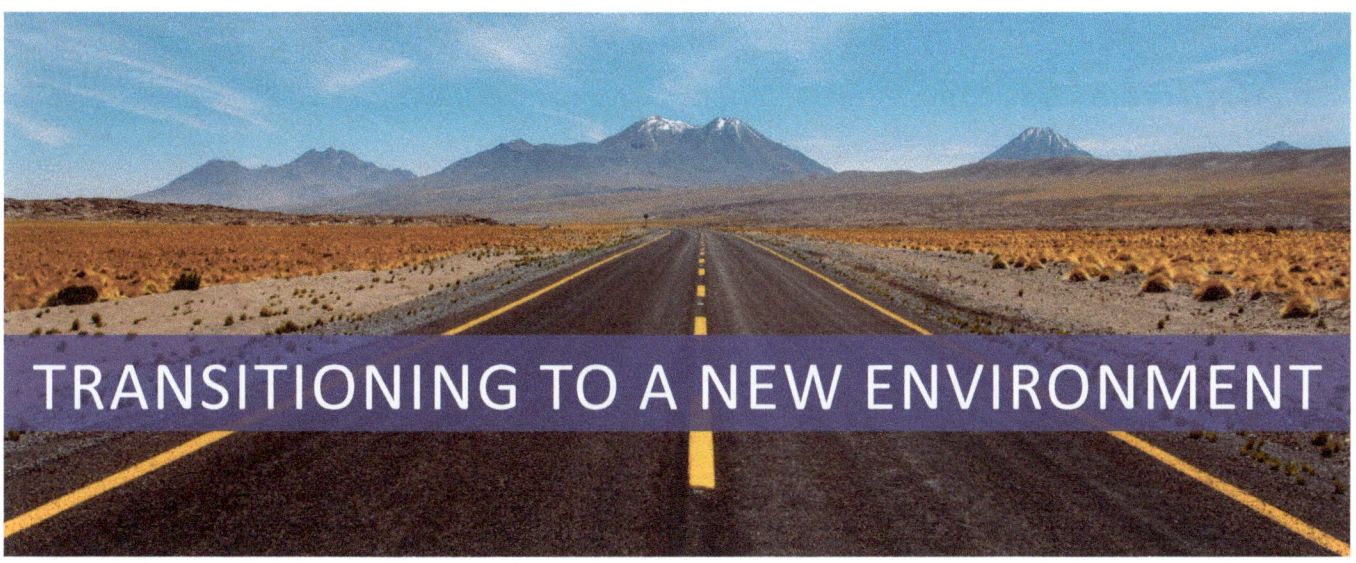

TRANSITIONING TO A NEW ENVIRONMENT

When entering a new environment, there may be new triggers for the child's meltdown. It is important for parents to work with teachers to find out what these triggers are and make the necessary adjustments to help the child adapt. For triggers that cannot be removed, the child should slowly be exposed to these triggers a bit at a time and eventually be able to function in school in the presence of these triggers.

For example, a child who is aversive to loud noises may find the national anthem during morning assembly overwhelming. Teachers can arrange for the student to stand away from the assembly area initially, gradually moving the child closer to the class at the assembly area.

⋯→ *Social stories*

Social stories are very important for a smoother transition to Primary 1. Parents are advised to read with the child the social stories every day. The social stories must include real-life pictures of the school compound.

Example 1: Going to primary one

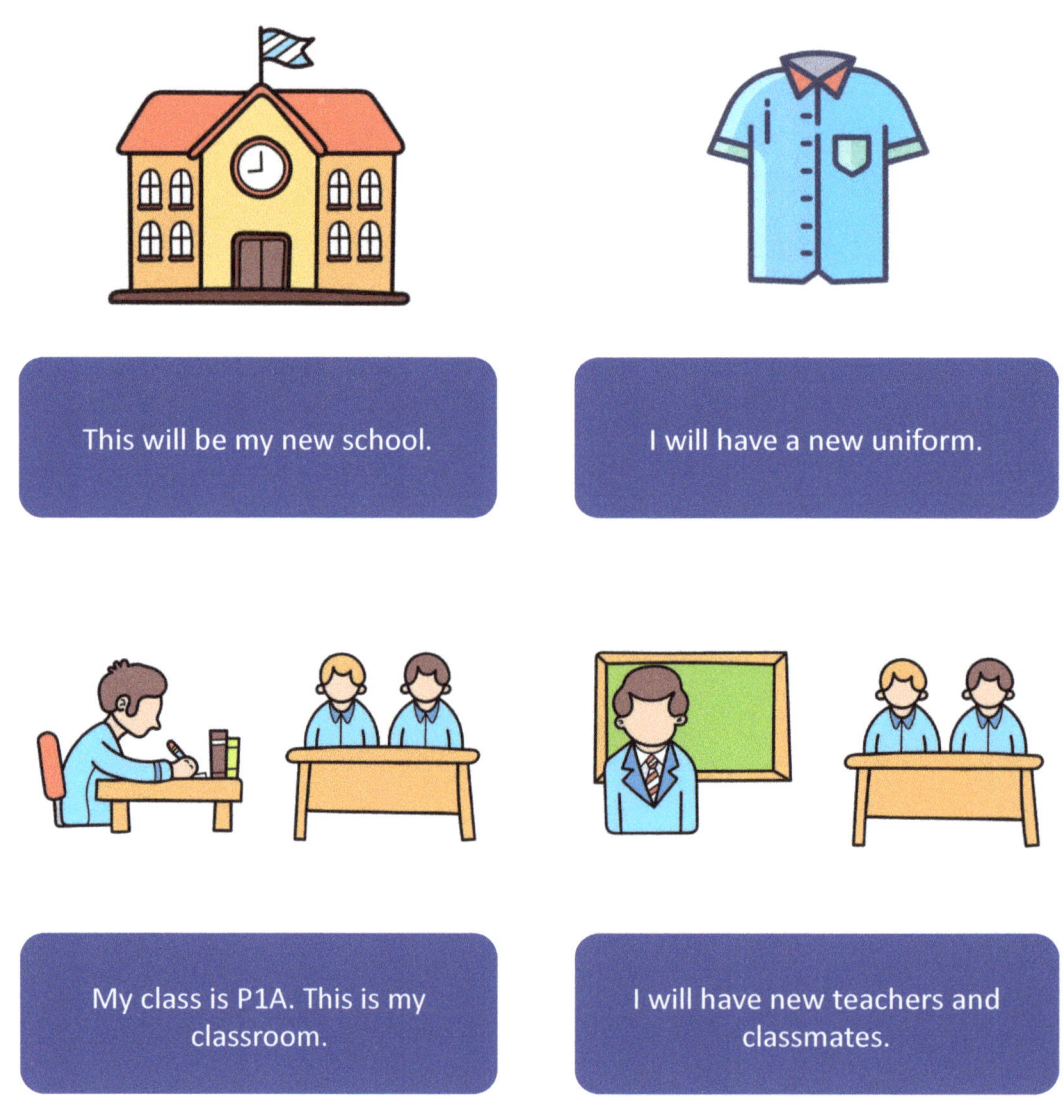

⋯→ *Social stories*

Example 1: Going to primary one (continued)

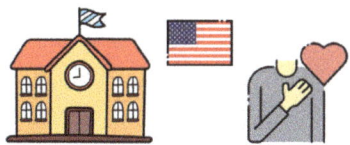  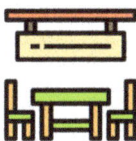  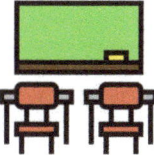

There wil be an assembly every morning. I will sing the National Anthem and take the pledge.

During school, I will also have "lunch time." During lunch time, I can have a break to rest, eat, or play with my friends.

When the bell rings, I must be back in my classroom and ready for the lesson to begin!

 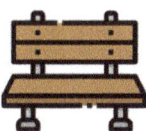  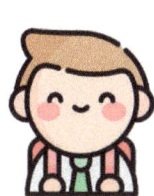 

There willl be an older schoolmate who will be my buddy. He or she will show me around my new school and tell me about the rules. I must listen to my buddy.

After school, I go to the benches to look for Mommy!

I am a very good student! I love going to school!

⤑ *Visual calendars*

Visual calendars can be used to count down with the child to the first day of Primary 1. Parents will get the child to cross out the date every day and point out to the child how many more days there are until important activities.

SUN	MON	TUES	WED	THURS	FRI	SAT
3 MARCH	4 X	5 X	6 X	7	8 ORIENTATION	9
10	11	12	13	14	15	16
17	18	19	20	21	22	23
24	25	26	27	28	29	30
31	1 APRIL	2 FIRST DAY OF P1	3	4	5	6

┈→ *Routines*

Parents should also prepare the child for important primary school routines such as the lunch routine, assembly routine, and work routine. Parents can roleplay the routines with the child to familiarize them before the commencement of school. More information on page 8.

	1	Think of what to buy
	2	Line up
	3	Order my food
	4	Pay money
	5	Take change
	6	Sit at table and eat

Example of a Lunch Routine

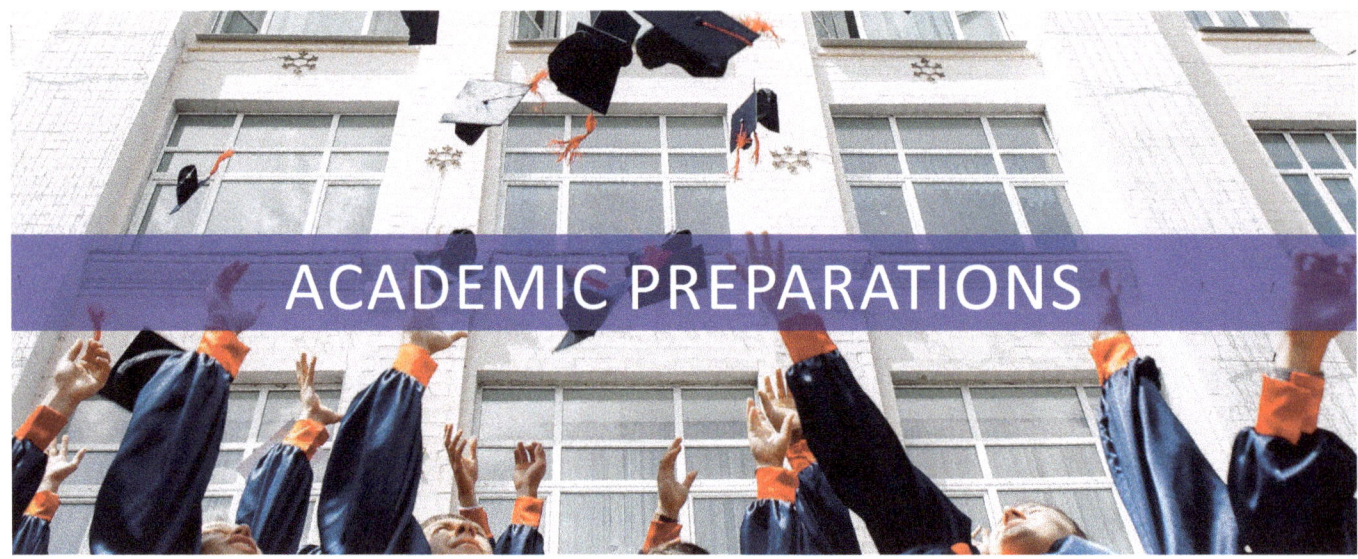

ACADEMIC PREPARATIONS

The jump from preschool to primary school may be stressful for the child. If possible, parents should try and teach the child the Primary 1 syllabus in advance to build up their confidence in primary school. This eventually helps the child understand lessons better and cope with the increasing academic demands. Parents can do this by:

→   **Working with the child regularly to train table habits and independent completion of tasks.**

→   **Looking through the Primary 1 syllabus, being aware of what the child will be learning, and guiding the child in those topics.**

→   **Working with school teachers to find out how to best help their child.**

BE PREPARED!

→ **Your child might take longer to transition to the new environment compared to other children. It is okay! Be patient and supportive— your child will adapt eventually!**

→ **Communicate constantly with your child's teachers! They are there to work with you to better support your child!**

→ **Stay calm and supportive. Your child can sense when you are anxious, and it may make them more anxious as well!**

→ **Praise your child after each successful day at school!**

APPENDIX

Appendix 1: Token economy (EIBI, Preschool)

Appendix 2: Task Schedule

Appendix 3: Token Economy (Primary School)

APPENDIX 1: Token Economy (EIBI, Preschool)

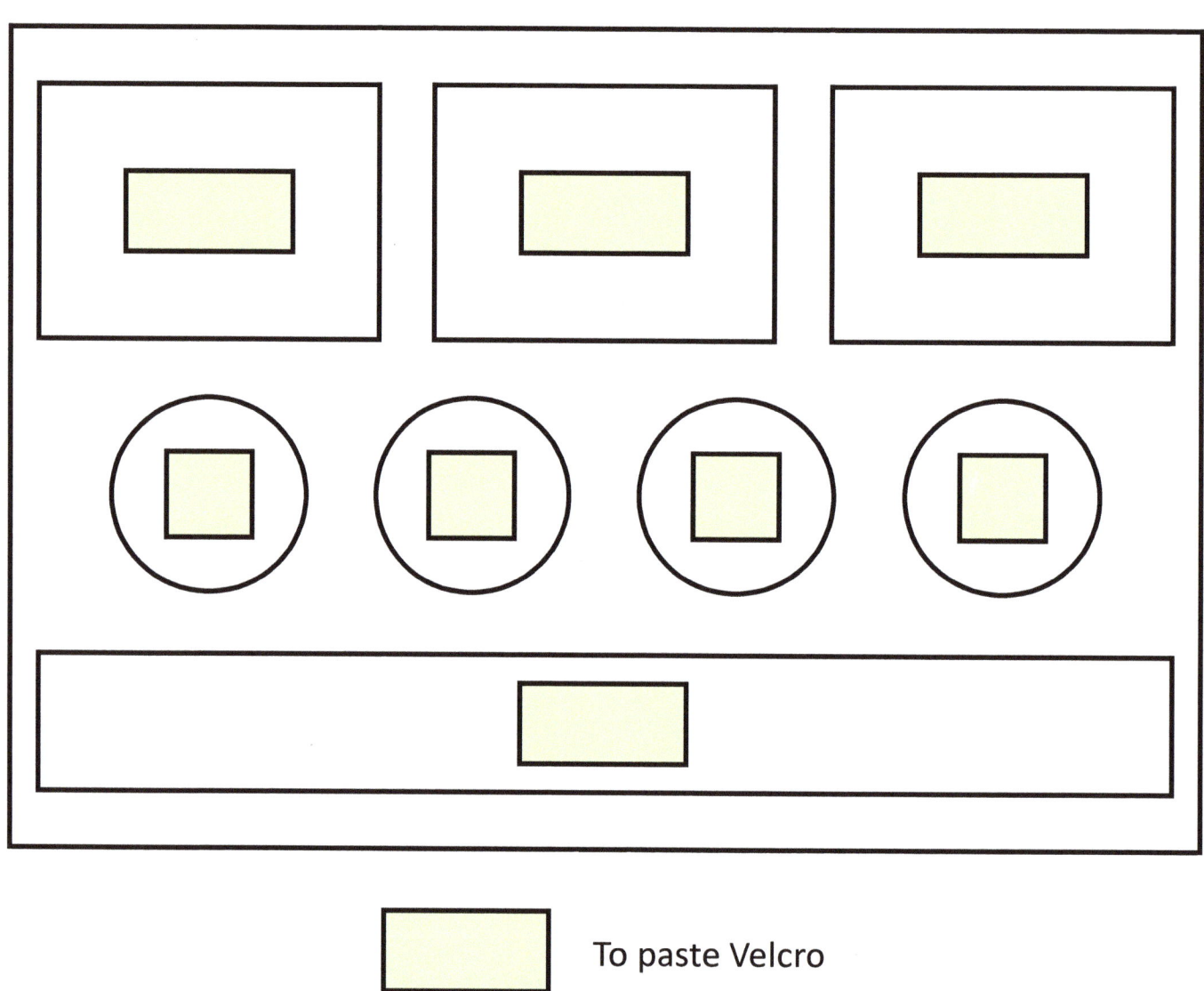

To paste Velcro

The following should be cut and laminated separately.

Tokens:

Reward strip:

Goals:

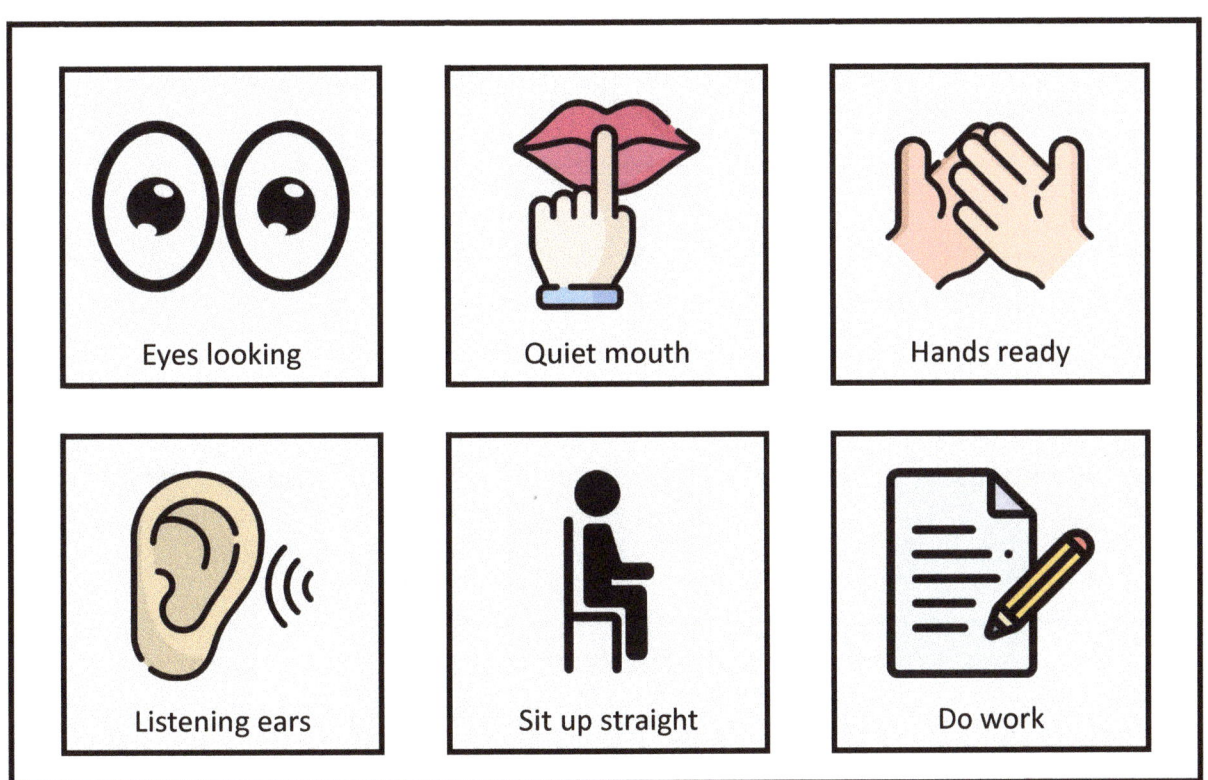

| Eyes looking | Quiet mouth | Hands ready |
| Listening ears | Sit up straight | Do work |

APPENDIX 2: Task Schedule

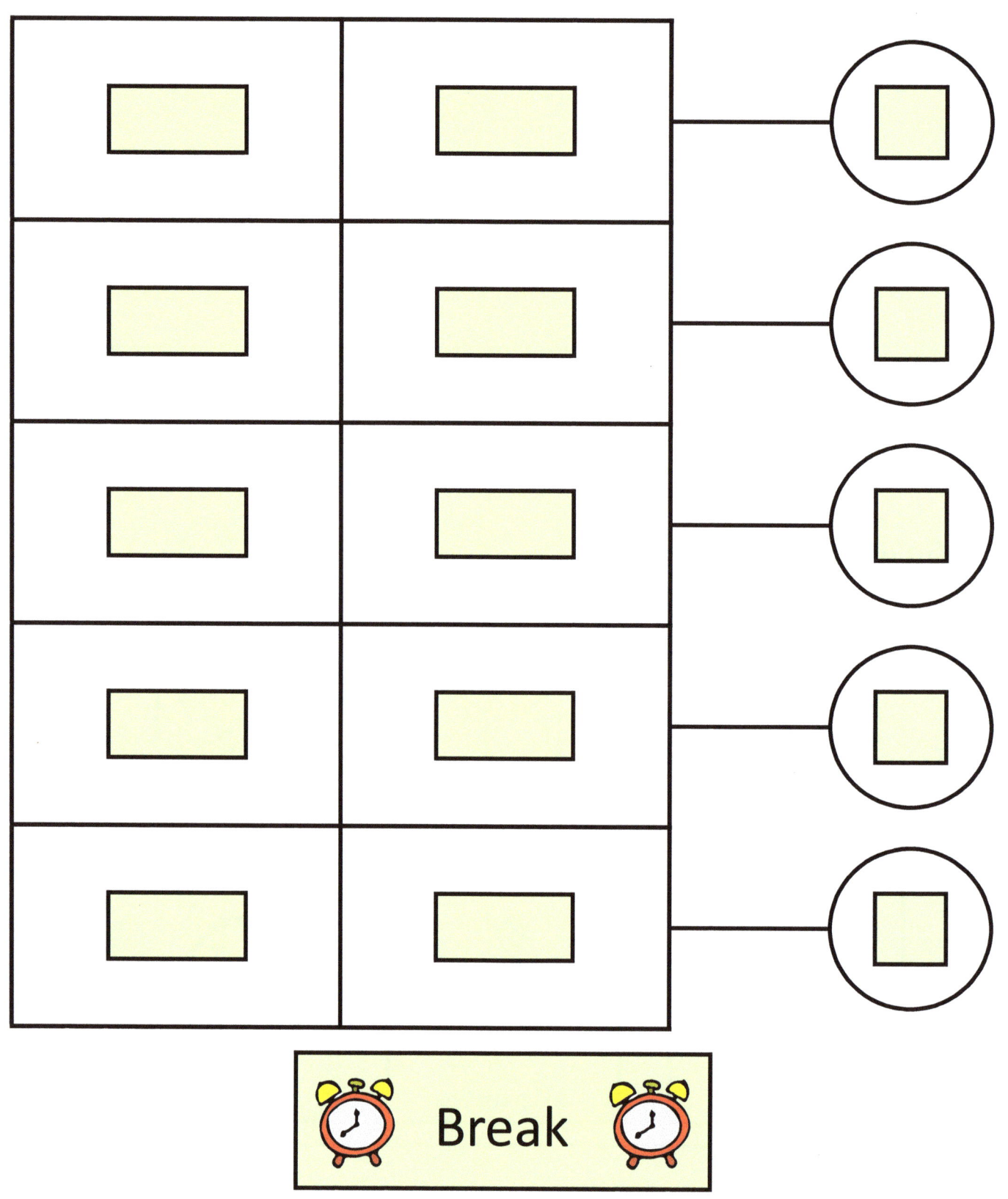

APPENDIX 2: Task Schedule

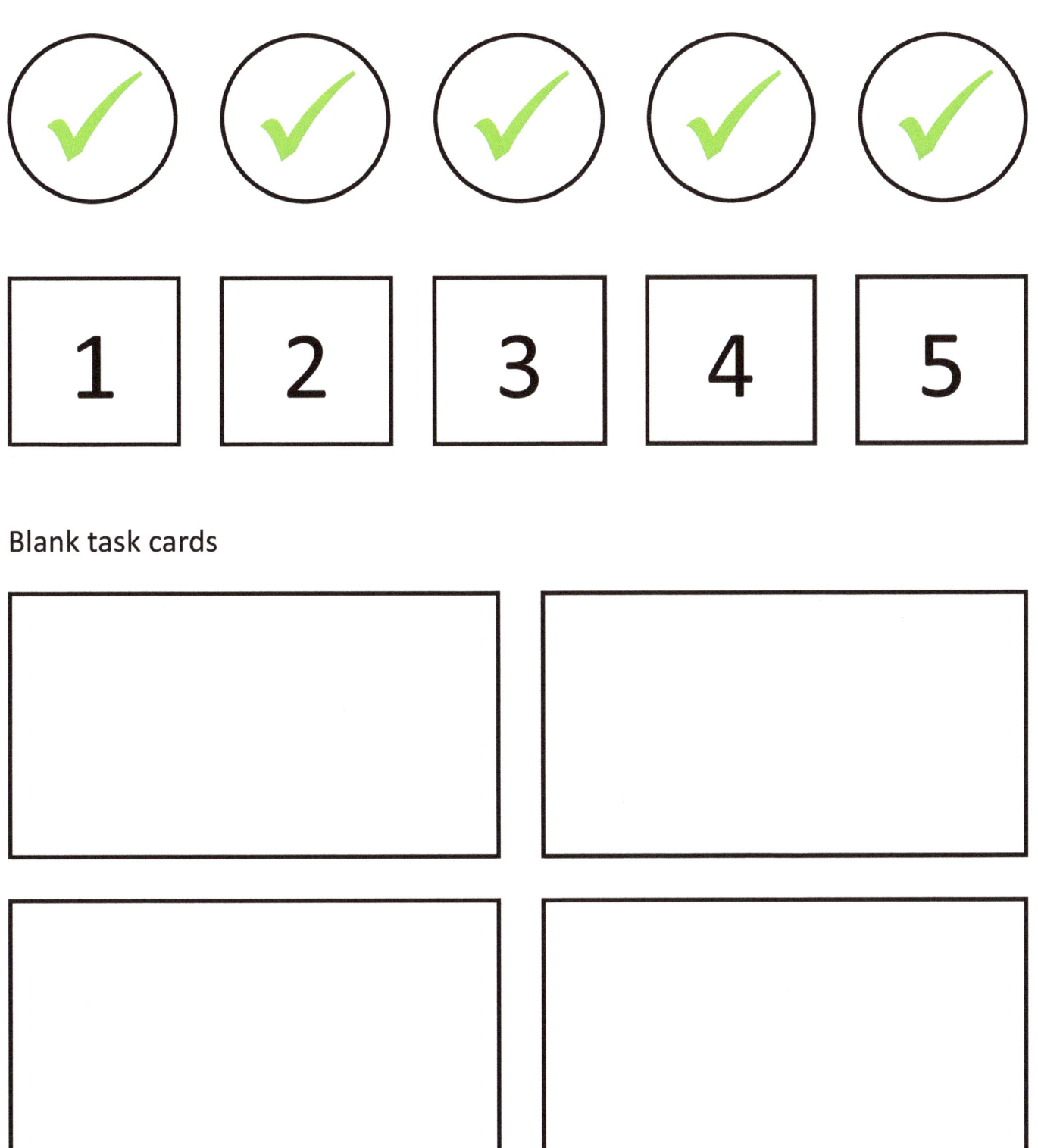

| 1 | 2 | 3 | 4 | 5 |

Blank task cards

APPENDIX 2: Task Schedule

Task card templates

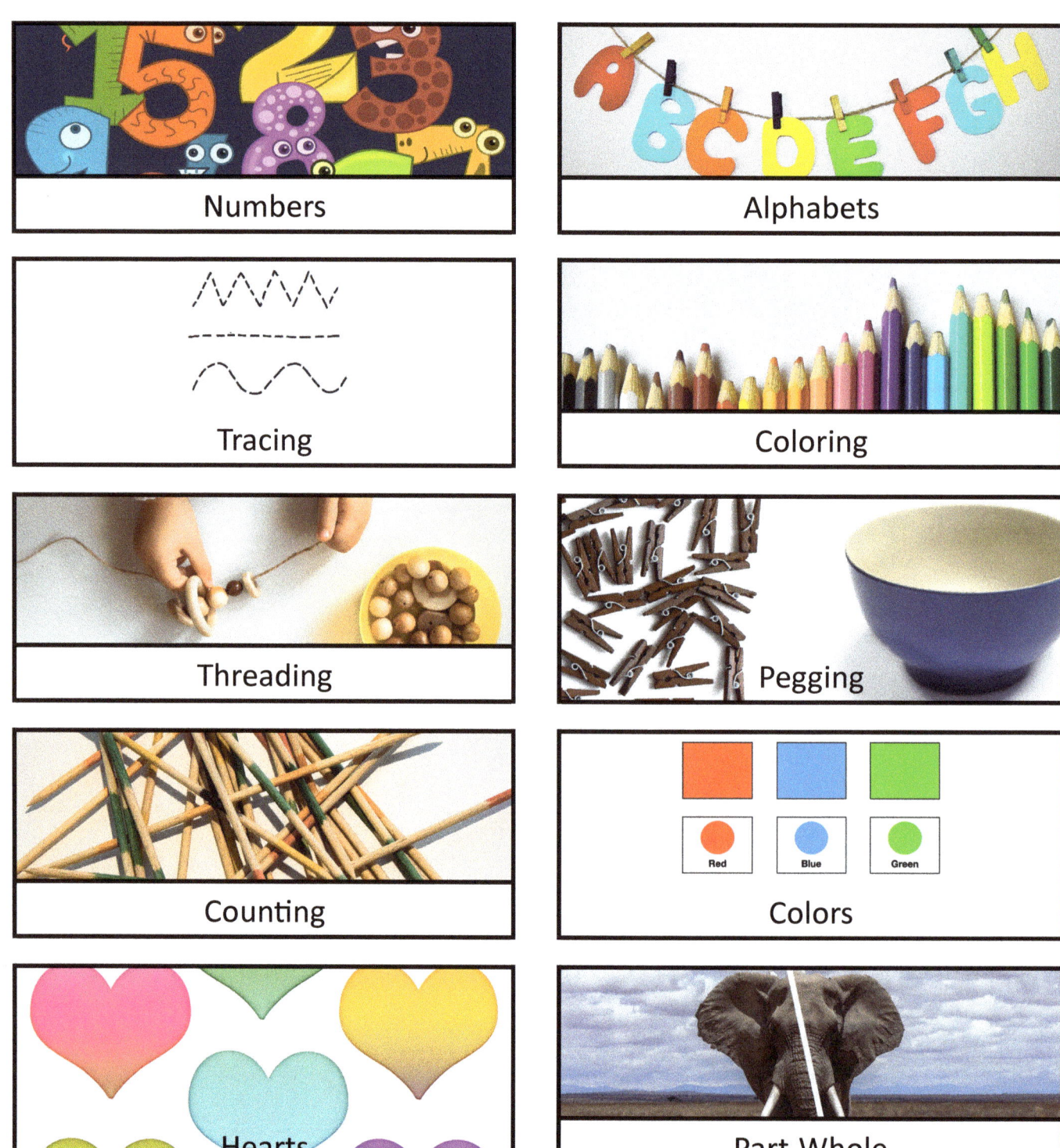

Numbers	Alphabets
Tracing	Coloring
Threading	Pegging
Counting	Colors
Hearts	Part-Whole

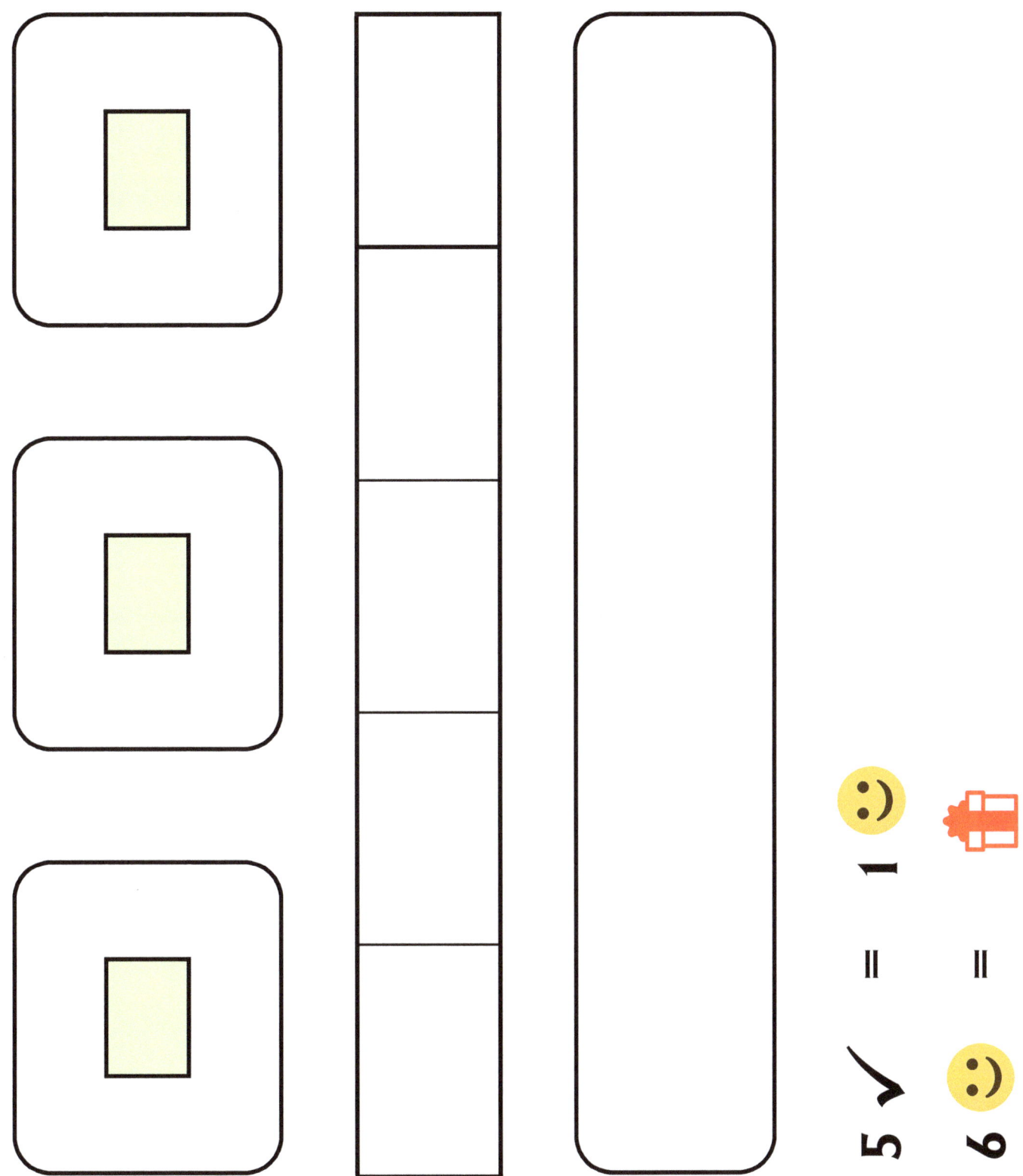

APPENDIX 3: Token Economy (Primary School)

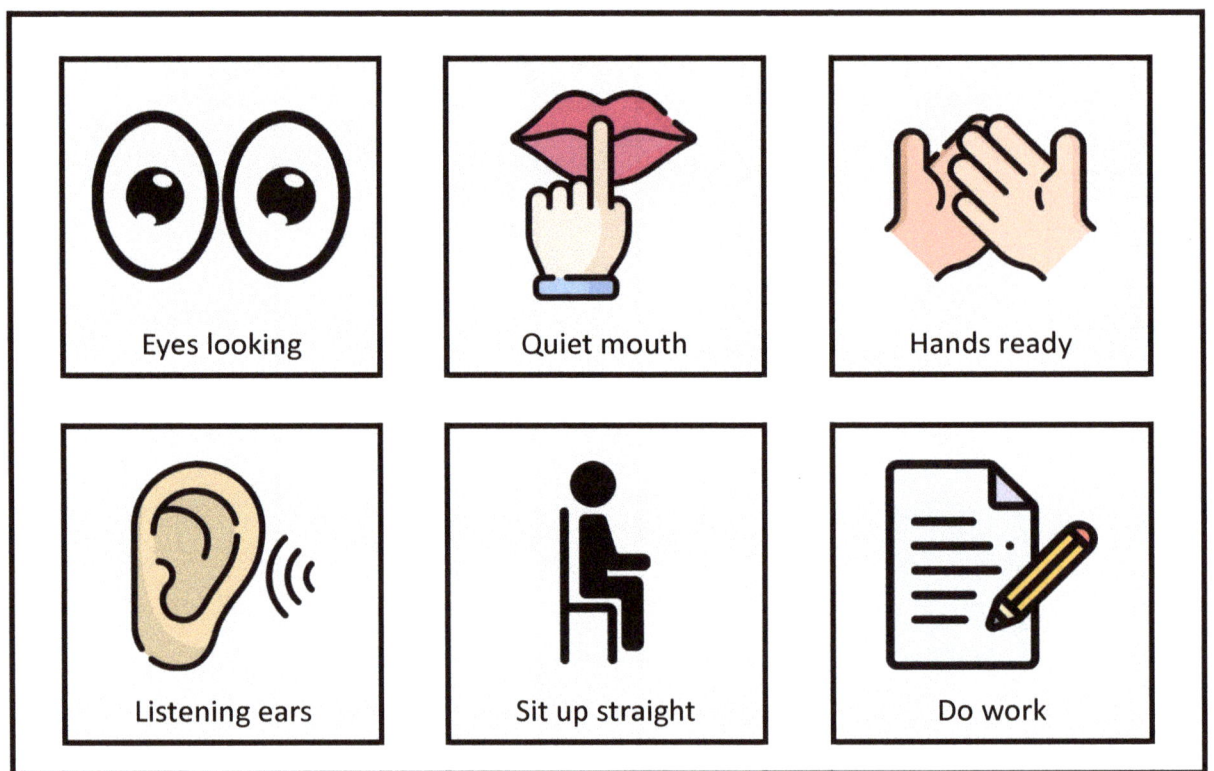

Other goal cards can be created based on child's needs:

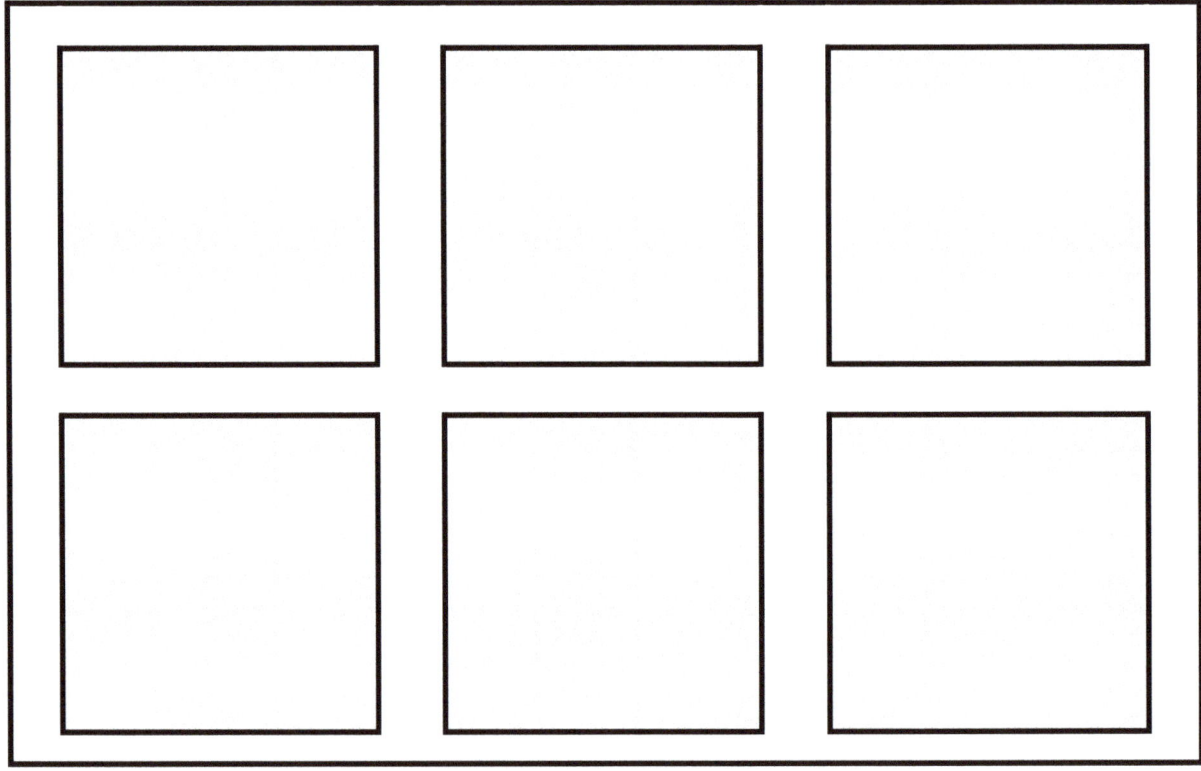

REFERENCES

Autism Speaks. "Study Finds Early Intervention Highly Effective." November 29, 2009. https://www.autismspeaks.org/science-news/early-intervention-toddlers-autism-highly-effective-study-finds.

Autism Speaks. "Autism Diagnostic Criteria: DSM 5." https://www.autismspeaks.org/autism-diagnosis-criteria-dsm-5.

Baker, Jed, and Alex Liau Whatt Meng. *School Shadow Guidelines*. Singapore: Nurture Pods Pte Ltd, 2014.

Burrell, T. Lindsey, and Joaquin Borrego, Jr. "Parents' Involvement in ASD Treatment: What is Their Role?" *Cognitive and Behavioral Practice* 19, no. 3 (2012): 423-432. doi: 10.1016/j.cbpra.2011.04.003.

Charlop-Christy, Marjorie H., Michael Carpenter, Loc Le, Kristen Kellet, and Linda Leblanc. "Using the Picture Exchange Communication System (PECS) with Children with Autism: Assessment of PECS Acquisition, Speech, Social-Communicative Behavior, and Problem Behavior." *Journal of Applied Behavior Analysis* 35, no. 3 (2002): 213-231. doi: 10.1901/jaba.2002.25-213.

Frost, Lori. "The Picture Exchange Communication System." *Perspectives on Language Learning and Education* 9, no. 2 (2002): 13-16. doi: 10.1044/lle9.2.13.

Ganz, Jennifer B., and Richard L. Simpson. "Effects on Communicative Requesting and Speech Development of the Picture Exchange Communication System in Children with Characteristics of Autism." *Journal of Autism and Developmental Disorders* 34, no. 4 (2004): 395-409. https://doi.org/10.1023/B:JADD.0000037416.59095.d7.

Goy, Priscilla, and Janice Tai. "1 in 150 Children in Singapore has Autism." The Straits Times. https://www.straitstimes.com/singapore/health/1-in-150-children-in-singapore-has-autism.

Kravits, Tamara R., Debra M. Kamps, Katie Kemmerer, and Jessica Potucek. "Brief Report: Increasing Communication Skills for an Elementary-Aged Student with Autism Using the Picture Exchange Communication System." *Journal of Autism and Developmental Disorders* 32, no. 3 (2002): 225-230. https://doi.org/10.1023/A:1015457932788.

Magiati, Iliana, and Patricia Howlin. "A Pilot Evaluation Study of the Picture Exchange Communication System (PECS) for Children with Autistic Spectrum Disorders." *Autism* 7, no. 3 (2003): 297-320. https://doi.org/10.1177/1362361303007003006.

Matson, Johnny L., and Jessica A. Boisjoli. "The Token Economy for Children with Intellectual Disability and/or Autism: A Review." *Research in Developmental Disabilities* 30, no. 2 (2009): 240-248. doi: 10.1016/j.ridd.2008.04.001.

National Autism Network. "Creating a Sensory Friendly Home Environment for Children on the Autism Spectrum." Office for People with Disabilities. https://www2.erie.gov/ecod/index.php?q=creating-sensory-friendly-home-environment-children-autism-spectrum.

National Institute of Mental Health. "Autism Spectrum Disorder." https://www.nimh.nih.gov/health/topics/autism-spectrum-disorders-asd/index.shtml.

Pickles, Andrew, Ann Le Couteur, Kathy Leadbitter, Erica Salomone, Rachel Cole-Fletcher, Hannah, Isobel Gammer, et al. Parent-Mediated Social Communication Therapy for Young Children with Autism (PACT): Long-Term Follow-Up of a Randomised Controlled Trial. *Lancet* 388, no. 10059 (2016): 2501-2509. https://doi.org/10.1016/S0140-6736(16)31229-6.

REFERENCES

Shapiro, Lawrence E. *101 Ways to Teach Children Social Skills: A Ready-to-Use, Reproducible Activity Book*. Plainview: The Bureau for At-Risk Youth.

Smith, Lori. (2018). "What is Stimming." Medical News Today. https://www.medicalnewstoday.com/articles/319714.

Tincani, Matt, Shannon Crozier, and Lindsay Alazetta. "The Picture Exchange Communication System: Effects on Manding and Speech Development for School-Aged Children with Autism." *Education and Training in Developmental Disabilities* 41, no. 2 (2006): 177-184. www.jstor.org/stable/23880179.

Warren, Zachary, Melissa L. McPheeters, Nila Sathe, Jennifer H. Foss-Feig, Allison Glasser, and Jeremy Veenstra-VanderWeele. "A Systematic Review of Early Intensive Intervention for Autism Spectrum Disorders." *Pediatrics* 127, no. 5 (2011): 1303-1311. doi: 10.1542/peds.2011-0426.

World Health Organization. "Autism Spectrum Disorders." World Health Organization. June 1, 2021. https://www.who.int/news-room/fact-sheets/detail/autism-spectrum-disorders.

CPSIA information can be obtained
at www.ICGtesting.com
Printed in the USA
LVHW022205071021
699864LV00001B/1